Breast and Nipple Pain

Edited by
Kathleen Kendall-Tackett, PhD, IBCLC, FAPA
& Scott Sherwood, BS

All royalties go to the
U.S. Lactation Consultant Association.

Praeclarus Press, LLC
©2015. United States Lactation Consultant Association

Praeclarus Press, LLC

2504 Sweetgum Lane

Amarillo, Texas 79124 USA

806-367-9950

www.PraeclarusPress.com

DISCLAIMER

The information contained in this publication is advisory only and is not intended to replace sound clinical judgment or individualized patient care. The author disclaims all warranties, whether expressed or implied, including any warranty as the quality, accuracy, safety, or suitability of this information for any particular purpose.

ISBN #978-1-939807-32-8

Cover Design: Ken Tackett

Acquisition & Development: Kathleen Kendall-Tackett & Scott Sherwood

Copy Editing: Kathleen Kendall-Tackett

Layout & Design: Nelly Murariu

Operations: Scott Sherwood

Contents

USLCA

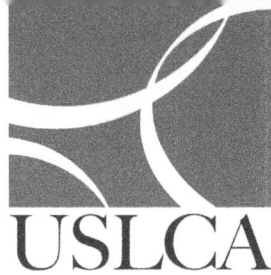

The Frequency and Resolution of Nipple Pain When Latch is Improved in a Private Practice

Véronique Darmangeat, IBCLC, RLC[1]

Keywords: Latch, lactation consultant private practice, breast pain, nipple pain

This study examined the frequency and resolution of nipple pain in 61 consecutive cases in a private practice. Out of 61 consultations, 37 mothers reported pain during feeds, either exclusively or combined with another problem. For 24 of these 37 mothers, the pain ended by improving the latch. For the 13 other mothers, there were additional problems associated with the pain that required further intervention. The majority of consultations for pain were resolved simply by improving the baby's positioning at the breast. This implies that it is important to address latch issues from the very first days of the baby's life.

1   veronique.darmangeat@wanadoo.fr. Article translated to English by Lea Cohen, IBCLC, leacohenibclc@gmail.com

Introduction

Nipple pain and inadequate weight gain are two common reasons for breastfeeding cessation. After leaving the maternity hospital, mothers often have difficulty finding help if they have breastfeeding problems. The author is an IBCLC in private practice who provides lactation support to families at any time during their breastfeeding experiences. The author noted that consultations frequently involved working with mothers to improve the babies' latch, with nipple pain as the presenting problem.

Given the frequency with which nipple pain and latch appeared to be the presenting problem, she sought to systematically evaluate the proportion of women seeking her services for nipple pain that could be improved simply by improving the baby's latch.

Method

The data included all consultation files from January 4, 2010 through February 22, 2010. This represented 59 cases and 61 consultations. All the cases were included, regardless of the age of the baby or the reason given by the mother for the consultation. All the mothers lived in France, in the region of Ile de France (the large region including and surrounding Paris). The consultations were conducted in the home ($n=49$), in the office ($n=10$), or by telephone ($n=2$).

The author asked each woman the following question during the consultation: *Do you feel pain when your baby latches on to the breast or during the feed?* The mothers' responses indicated whether pain was their presenting problem, either exclusively or combined with another problem. In all the cases of pain, the baby's latch was evaluated and the mother was offered suggestions for improving the baby's positioning at the breast. The pain was re-evaluated after latch improvement. The absence of pain was the criteria for saying that simple improvement of the latch was sufficient to resolve the pain problem. For each mother-baby couple, latch difficulties, and any of the other problems that might have led to pain at latching, were noted. This information was included in the mother's file, and data for this study were coded from the mothers' files.

Results

The age of the babies seen in consultation varied from 4 days old to one year. The average age was 32 days. Sixty-two percent of the 61 consultations were for breast pain. Pain may have been the only reason given for the consultation, or there may have been another problem, such as an insufficient weight gain, mastitis, problems with the feeding rhythm, or premature weaning.

Many of these issues are linked to breast pain because a baby who hurts his mother when breastfeeding may have an inefficient suck, which can lead to inadequate weight gain. The baby's inability to empty the breasts sufficiently can lead to mastitis, and the baby might nurse continuously to build up an inadequate milk supply. All of these problems can lead to premature weaning. The consultations for pain represented almost two thirds of the author's consultations during these two months. Some women waited several months, and one of them a whole year, before consulting because they had been told at the maternity hospital that it was normal to have breast pain during breastfeeding.

Sixty-five percent of the breast-pain cases resolved simply by improving the latch of the baby. In all these cases, the mothers declared that it was the first time that they had been shown how to offer their breast to their babies in a way that didn't hurt.

Thirty-five percent of the pain cases associated with an incorrect latch co-occurred with another problem.

These problems included:

» Dermatological conditions, such as eczema or sebaceous cyst

» Short lingual frenulum

» Jaw problems, including hypertonicity of the jaw, or asymmetrical jaws

» Candidiasis

» Bacterial infection in the breast

» Sucking problem in the baby

In all these cases, it was necessary to treat both the baby's latch and the other causes of the pain.

The most common latch issues were as follows:

» The baby did not open his mouth sufficiently. The nipple was centered in the baby's mouth, or the upper lip was not being stimulated.

» The baby opened his mouth correctly, but then shut it because he was held too far from the breast. The baby had to lower his head to take the breast, the mother bent forward to bring the baby to the breast, or the mother pressed on the chin of the baby.

» The baby turned his head to take the breast because the mother positioned him with his stomach facing upwards, often by placing him on a breast-feeding pillow that was not the right height.

To help these babies latch onto the breast without provoking pain, two positions were used by the author, depending on the case.

» Placing the baby in the cross-cradle position, as described by Dr. Jack Newman and Teresa Pitman (2006). The baby is held tightly against the mother's body, stomach to stomach, his head is in a slight backwards extension and his chin touches the breast first. The mouth is wide open and the nipple is directed towards the upper lip.

» The Biological Nurturing™ position as described by Dr. Suzanne Colson (2005; 2008; 2011). The mother is in a semi-lying or semi-sitting, laid-back position. The baby is placed stomach to stomach on his mother and can use his feet to direct himself towards the breast. His head is in a slight backwards extension and the baby opens his mouth very wide to take in the breast.

For women using a breastfeeding pillow, the author suggested that they either abandon it, or use a firm pillow that is placed high enough to allow the baby to be at breast height.

Discussion

Nipple pain was a common problem reported by mothers in this private practice. This study is small and the results cannot be generalized to all private practices without further research. Nevertheless, it is interesting to note that all the women suffering from pain when latching on—whose pains were resolved by improving the latch—reported that they had not received prior assistance in latching the baby in a way that did not cause pain. Each of these women was seen by the author subsequent to their stay in the maternity ward.

In addition, it can be noted that helping mothers improve their latch represents the essential work of the author's practice. These findings suggest that there is a lack of information given to mothers in the hospital. This could be due to personnel that are insufficiently trained, limited time spent with mothers (usually due to a lack of personnel in the hospital), and limited number of lactation consultants in French hospitals. Further, hospital personnel may believe that they have given the information to the mother, but the mother may not have understood or really received it.

In a certain number of cases, the women who came to consult had already consulted with other healthcare providers for these pains, and were treated for a yeast or bacterial infection, or they had been told to clip a baby's tongue-tie, without verifying and improving the latch. In all these cases, these first treatment attempts were ineffectual because the underlying problem, the inadequate latch, was not addressed.

Further, it must be noted that French women do not have easy access to correct photos or drawings of appropriate latch. The photos used in publications about breastfeeding mostly show babies taking the breast without properly opening their mouth.

Since most women have never seen a breastfed baby in their circle of acquaintances, they no longer receive this information via informal, mother-to-mother channels and must rely upon maternity personnel. However, three days spent in the maternity hospital cannot replace the saturation of information they would have received during childhood had they grown up in a breastfeeding culture.

Conclusion

A good latch is essential to assure a comfortable and effective feed. This latch should be shown to women in such a way that they are capable of replicating it once they are alone with their babies. This type of support takes time and mothers do not always get it. Therefore, lactation consultants in private practice have an important role to play in providing this type of support for mothers. The majority of the author's consultations are focused on improving the latch. A future study can address pain management in breastfeeding women on a larger scale.

References

Colson, S.D. (2005). Maternal breastfeeding position: Have we got it right? *Practising Midwife*, 8(10), 24, 26-7, 29-32.

Colson, S.D. (2011). *Biological nurturing: Laid-back breastfeeding for mothers.* Pasadena, CA: Geddes Productions.

Colson, S.D., Meek, J.H., & Hawdon, J.M. (2008). Optimal positions for the release of primitive neonatal reflexes stimulating breastfeeding. *Early Human Development*, 84(7), 441-449.

Newman, J., & Pitman, T. (2006). *L'allaitement:comprendre et réussir.* Toronto : Jack Newman Communications.

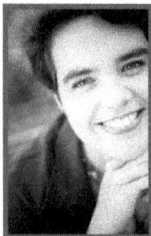

Véronique Darmangeat, IBCLC, RLC, is a lactation consultant in France, founder of the firm, Lactissima, and writes the blog, *A tire d'Ailes*. She does consultations, and trains, writes books, and gives lectures.

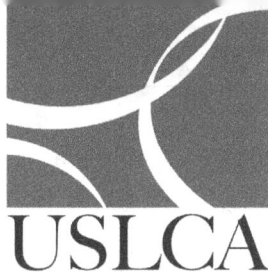

Raynaud's Phenomenon, Candidiasis, and Nipple Pain
Strategies for Differential Diagnosis and Care

Genae D. Strong, Ph.D., CNM, RNC-OB, IBCLC, RLC[1]
Nancy Mele, DSN, RN[2]

Keywords: Nipple pain, Raynaud's, vasospasm, breastfeeding

Breastfeeding pain is the second most common reason women stop breastfeeding (Strong, 2011); therefore it should be recognized early and treated promptly. Often pain from primary Raynaud's Phenomenon of the Nipple (RP-n) imitates Candidiasis, misleading providers who prescribe antifungal medications. Unfortunately, the correct diagnosis comes after multiple doses of medication and no improvement in breastfeeding pain. Antifungals can further complicate diagnosis because they can cause nipple vasospasm as a side-effect of treatment (Bonyata, 2011). This article presents a case study of RP-n mistaken for Candidiasis. Evidenced-based treatment strategies, education, and close follow-up are minimum standards of care for women with breastfeeding pain.

1 gdstrong@memphis.edu
2 nmele@memphis.edu

Fragmented healthcare systems can interfere with coordinated, evidence-based care. Raynaud's and Candidiasis can present in very similar manners resulting in a clinical dilemma for providers. However, excellent systematic clinical assessment focusing on the characteristics of the pain can help to differentiate between the two conditions. An algorithm to assist providers in differentiating between the two has been developed.

Breastfeeding is being recognized as the healthiest infant feeding method. Unfortunately, difficulties encountered during a breastfeeding experience can have an enduring effect on both the current breastfeeding relationship and attitudes about further attempts (La Leche League International, 2008). Timely resolution of problems is essential if nursing mothers are to achieve their breastfeeding goals.

A nurse is often the first and in some cases the only provider to assist new mothers with breastfeeding during the perinatal period. As the largest part of the healthcare team, nurses play a critical role in educating, assisting, and supporting breastfeeding families. In addition, nurses ensure continuity of care by collaborating and/or referring women for complex breastfeeding situations to professionals certified in the clinical management of breastfeeding and human lactation, International Board Certified Lactation Consultants (IBCLCs). This positions both the nurse and the IBCLC as primary interventionists in preventing and solving breastfeeding problems and challenges (Walker, 2008).

Unresolved problems are likely to lead to early weaning and feelings of failure that can influence subsequent feeding decisions (McClellan et al., 2012). This case study presents the clinical dilemma associated with the assessment, diagnosis, and treatment of nipple pain and vasospasm associated with Raynaud's Phenomenon of the nipple (RP-n). Nipple pain, blanching, and vasospasm can be related to nipple compression or trauma and should be considered during assessment. We will briefly consider these conditions as part of this clinical dilemma. But the focus of this discussion is on the assessment of nipple pain related to RP-n or Candidiasis to further educate clinicians on how to identify and treat these two problems.

Nipple Blanching and Vasospasm

When the blood flow to the nipple is decreased or cut off temporarily the nipple may turn white, a condition known as nipple blanching. This most often occurs after a feeding and can be, but is not always, associated with pain (Walker, 2008). The nipple is usually white or pale and misshapen after coming out of the infant's mouth. If there is pain, it will occur seconds after nursing as the circulation is restored. The principal problem associated with nipple blanching is mechanical in nature and correcting a poor latch resulting in nipple compression is the first-line treatment choice. Assessment should include contributing factors, such as clamping due to rapid let-down, tongue-tie, or palate variations (Bonyata, 2011).

When blood vessels in the nipple constrict suddenly causing pain after nursing, or in between feedings, this is a more serious condition known as vasospasm. This condition can be extremely painful for some and not painful for others. Vasospasm can occur in conjunction with other causes of pain, or alone, but most likely from damaged nipples or Candidiasis (Newman & Kernerman, 2009).

Unlike blanching, positioning and latch are not implicated. Healing the nipple trauma should resolve this condition unless the underlying cause is part of a larger syndrome, such as Raynaud's Phenomenon (Australian Breastfeeding Association, 2011; Bonyata, 2011; Goldfarb, 2002-2011).

Raynaud's Phenomenon

Raynaud's Phenomenon (RP) is a vasospastic disorder associated with exposure to cold temperatures or stress resulting in a decreased blood supply to the outer extremities, generally the hands and feet. More specifically, hyperactivation of the sympathetic system causes extreme vasoconstriction of peripheral arteries and arterioles resulting in tissue hypoxia. The pathophysiology is not completely understood and may be multi-factorial, including vascular, intravascular, and neural mediators (Levien, 2010).

Characteristically there is a biphasic or triphasic color change in the affected areas, from white (pallor) to blue (hypoxia) to red (hyperemia), accompanied by numbness, tingling, and pain. When the episode subsides, or the area is warmed, color returns to normal. Not all patients experience color changes associated with classic RP, especially in milder cases. The cyclic color changes of classic RP may disappear during pregnancy because of increased surface blood flow. In nursing mothers, the nipples usually turn white and can be very painful. This phenomenon can be idiopathic (Raynaud's Disease/Primary RP) or associated with a wide variety of other conditions (Raynaud's Syndrome/Secondary RP).

Primary RP may be the first presenting symptom of diseases associated with Secondary RP, making this condition an important part of the documented health history (U.S. Department of Health & Human Services, 2011).

Raynaud's Phenomenon affects 20% of all women of childbearing age (O'Sullivan & Keith, 2011). Although RP was first described in 1862, the relationship between nipple vasospasm and RP was not suggested until 1992 (Morino & Winn, 2007). Many practicing clinicians are unaware of this condition and mistake it for Candidiasis. The literature suggests using a bacteriological analysis of breast milk to differentially diagnose Raynaud's syndrome from other infectious conditions (Delgado et al., 2009). Cultures will be negative in RP-n. However, this study was done with a small sample of 10 lactating women, five with RP-n and five with mastitis. Further research is needed to substantiate this as a valuable diagnostic tool.

In multiple case studies of RP-n that appeared in the literature between 1997 and 2007, the majority of women received antifungal therapy without relief before a diagnosis of RP-n was made. Anecdotal evidence from multiple breastfeeding blog sites indicates that clinicians remain unfamiliar with this condition and may not take it seriously (Hills, 2011; Hoen & Backe, 2009; Sealy, 2011; Yetter, 2011).

Raynaud's Phenomenon of the nipple is a condition that can frequently be managed by avoiding triggers. Normal behaviors associated with breastfeeding, like offering a wet nipple to encourage latch, wearing breast pads that become wet when milk lets down, and feeding during colder nighttime hours, can contribute to vasospasm. High levels of estrogen have also been implicated because of estrogen's association with the body's reaction to cold (Hills, 2011).

Other triggers that have been identified include stress, caffeine consumption, smoking, alcohol, and medications that promote vasoconstriction. Women should be instructed to avoid lifestyle triggers, reduce emotional stress, and avoid sudden temperature change or cold environments. Wearing warm clothing and keeping the ambient temperature warm can prevent episodes of vasospasm (Anderson et al., 2004; Bonyata, 2011; Morino & Winn, 2007). Taking a warm shower or applying dry heat to the breast after breastfeeding is also suggested as a method of alleviating discomfort (Riordan & Wambach, 2010). Drinking a hot beverage can also help, as it raises core body temperature.

When prevention is unsuccessful there are a variety of supplements, herbs, and drugs that can be used to control the discomfort associated with this condition. There is evidence to suggest that dietary supplementation with calcium and magnesium or vitamin B_6, evening primrose oil, olive oil, or fish oil can reduce symptoms (Anderson et al., 2004; Newman & Kernerman, 2009). The medical alternative to complementary therapies is the use of a calcium channel blocker, like nifedipine. These medications inhibit the uptake of calcium by vascular smooth muscles resulting in vasodilation (Garrison, 2002). .

Candidiasis

Candidiasis is an overgrowth of naturally occurring yeast, *Candida albicans*, which lives on the skin, and the mucous membranes, and the genitourinary track. Because the infant's mouth and mother's nipples are warm and moist, this yeast readily grows in these areas. Candidiasis can occur at any time during lactation, but infants or mothers who have received antibiotic therapy, or mothers with nipple trauma, are more susceptible.

Additionally, mothers with vaginal Candidiasis prior to delivery can infect their infants during vaginal birth, who then infect the mothers' breast and nipple during breastfeeding (Brent, 2001; Riordan & Wambach, 2010). Organism transfer has been significantly associated with the use of pacifiers and bottles containing artificial milk fortified with iron (Morrill et al., 2005) or high levels of sugars. Diagnosing this condition can be problematic because it is based on history, physical examination, and clinical symptoms rather than a laboratory test. There is ongoing controversy in the literature regarding whether *Candida albicans* can reside in the ductal system of the breast and play a significant role in breast pain and infection (Amir et al., 2011; Delgado et al., 2009; Hale et al., 2009).

Several studies have attempted to confirm diagnosis with milk and nipple cultures. But the accuracy and methodologies are highly contentious. Lactoferrin, which is present in human milk, inhibits growth of *Candida*. *Candida albicans* is a common fungus colonized in human tissues, and as many as 80 to 90 percent of infants have culturable *Candida albicans* present in their mouths. Another difficulty in using cultures to diagnose *Candida* is that mothers continue to be in pain while waiting on lab results.

Less disputable is the necessity for early recognition and treatment utilizing excellent systematic clinical skills. Typical symptoms given by mothers with presumptive Candidiasis are persistent sore nipples; rapid development of soreness; flaky, red, shiny skin; burning or itching; and shooting or stabbing pains deep into the breast. Mothers usually complain of severe discomfort and tenderness during or immediately after feedings. However, complaints of pain may not present exactly as described.

Assessing and correcting for mechanical abnormalities as well as ruling out pathophysiological reasons, such as vasospasms and Raynaud's phenomenon, are first-line treatment approaches. Other interventions include air drying nipples, disposing of wet nursing pads, wearing 100% cotton bras and underwear that can be washed in very hot water, making dietary changes, and taking acidophilus daily for two weeks beyond symptoms (Riordan & Wambach, 2010).

There are a number of treatment options that have not proven effective, such as applying warm wet compresses, tea bags, and oils. First-line pharmacologic treatments include mupirocin 2% ointment, clotrimazole topical antifungal applied in very thin coats to the nipple. Gentian violet kills *Candida* and can be painted on the nipples and areolae. Miconazole gel can be used for the infant's mouth and can be applied after each feeding.

When all other measures fail and/or culture results confirm *Candida* in the milk, Fluconazole can be used. Fluconazole is a systemic agent that can be used until the mother is relieved from pain. Treatment strategies should occur simultaneously by using pharmacological and nonpharmacological interventions as well as treating mother and infant.

Although Candidiasis is often diagnosed in breastfeeding women presenting with breast pain, other microorganisms have been implicated in breast infection and should not be overlooked.

Milk cultures have identified the presence of both *staphylococcus aureus* (s-au) and *streptococcus*. The presence of these two bacteria does not predict a breast infection unless there are other risk factors, such as cracked nipples or a previous mastitis. Cracked nipples potentiate a point of entry for both bacteria and *Candida*. These findings question antifungals as a first-line treatment without laboratory confirmation (Betzold, 2012; Hale et al., 2009). Evidenced-based treatment strategies, education, and close follow-up are minimum standards of care for women with breastfeeding pain. Candidiasis can lead to frustration in the breastfeeding mother if pain is not relieved.

Healthcare providers should encourage women to continue breastfeeding even though they may not get immediate relief. Good documentation is essential to mapping the progression and treatment efforts especially for those women who are more susceptible to Candidiasis.

Case Presentation

LM was a 30-year old first time mother with a pregnancy complicated by pre-eclampsia and postpartum hemorrhage. Her delivery was induced at 38 weeks following elevated blood pressures and uric acid levels in the presence of a ripe cervix. She delivered a healthy male child with APGAR scores of 9 and 10. LM was a healthcare provider who worked in the same metropolitan hospital where she delivered.

She was committed to early and exclusive breastfeeding and was well prepared for a natural childbirth experience with a doula in attendance. She also attended a breastfeeding workshop prior to delivery. Breastfeeding began with skin-to-skin contact immediately following delivery and continued on demand with rooming-in during a three-day hospital stay.

While in the hospital, LM experienced nipple pain that increased with each subsequent feeding. The two physicians who saw her and the baby in the hospital both supported her desire to breastfeed, but provided no breastfeeding assessment, support, or referral.

The nurses provided her with nipple shields for the pain, but never did a breast, latch, or feeding assessment. Lactation consultant services were not available over the weekend when she delivered. She quickly lost confidence in the nursing staff and believed they didn't know any more than she did.

> They knew what I knew ... If I had to say one word it would be nurses are clueless.

Therefore, LM was discharged with breast pain without a referral to an IBCLC or community resources. At one week postpartum, LM encountered a friend who was a lactation consultant (IBCLC). The IBCLC evaluated her latch and identified a disorganized sucking pattern requiring tongue training. After LM taught the infant to suck, the nipple pain subsided temporarily, but at five weeks she still felt sharp, shooting, tingling pain from the top of the breast to the nipple. She also noticed *white patches* on the nipples. Several weeks later, the pediatrician noticed a white patch in the infant's mouth and diagnosed him with thrush. During the interval between these two events, LM received a 10-day course of antibiotics. Nystatin Suspension was prescribed for the infant. The obstetrician was notified and requested nipple cultures for yeast, which proved to be negative. At the same visit an oral antifungal and topical cream were prescribed for her. The infant responded well to treatment, but the mother continued to experience pain.

By 12 weeks, LM received four rounds of antifungal therapy without relief. At this point she feared she would be forced to stop breastfeeding because she was returning to work and needed to pump.

> I hope this doesn't make me quit, not because of the medication, but because of the pumping factor...you can't pump when you have yeast....I was very upset that I had yeast that I couldn't get rid of and I had to pump!

In frustration LM called her friend, the IBCLC, and arranged for a consultation during which RP-n was noted on assessment.

> After everything didn't work, she looked at it and said that looks like Raynaud's.

Nifedipine was discussed as a first-line treatment, but LM, who had a past medical history of low blood pressure, was afraid to take it because of the rapid lowering of blood pressure associated with its use. She continued to breast-feed for thirteen months, pumping while at work, and using warm compresses on the nipple to manage the pain.

I found it to be a good experience even though some crazy things happened. I know a lot more now....I would do it again, I did do it again.

LM has subsequently had a second pregnancy and successfully breastfed this infant also.

Discussion

Breastfeeding support should occur across the perinatal experience. This case illuminates serious issues with the current healthcare system and quality of healthcare provided to breastfeeding women in the hospital and beyond. As we have established earlier, breastfeeding pain is a common reason women stop breastfeeding or decide not to begin.

Mothers need support, encouragement, and close follow-up, particularly during the hospital stay and after discharge to promote continuation of breastfeeding. The hospital nurses failed LM because they did not adequately assist her with basic breastfeeding care, nor did they initiate a referral to an IBCLC for a comprehensive assessment prior to leaving the hospital. Problems that should have been identified and addressed early went unresolved, resulting in nipple trauma, unnecessary treatments, and undiagnosed RP-n. LM was very committed to breastfeeding despite the challenges she encountered. However, a less-dedicated mother with fewer informal healthcare resources would likely have given up in the face of these challenges.

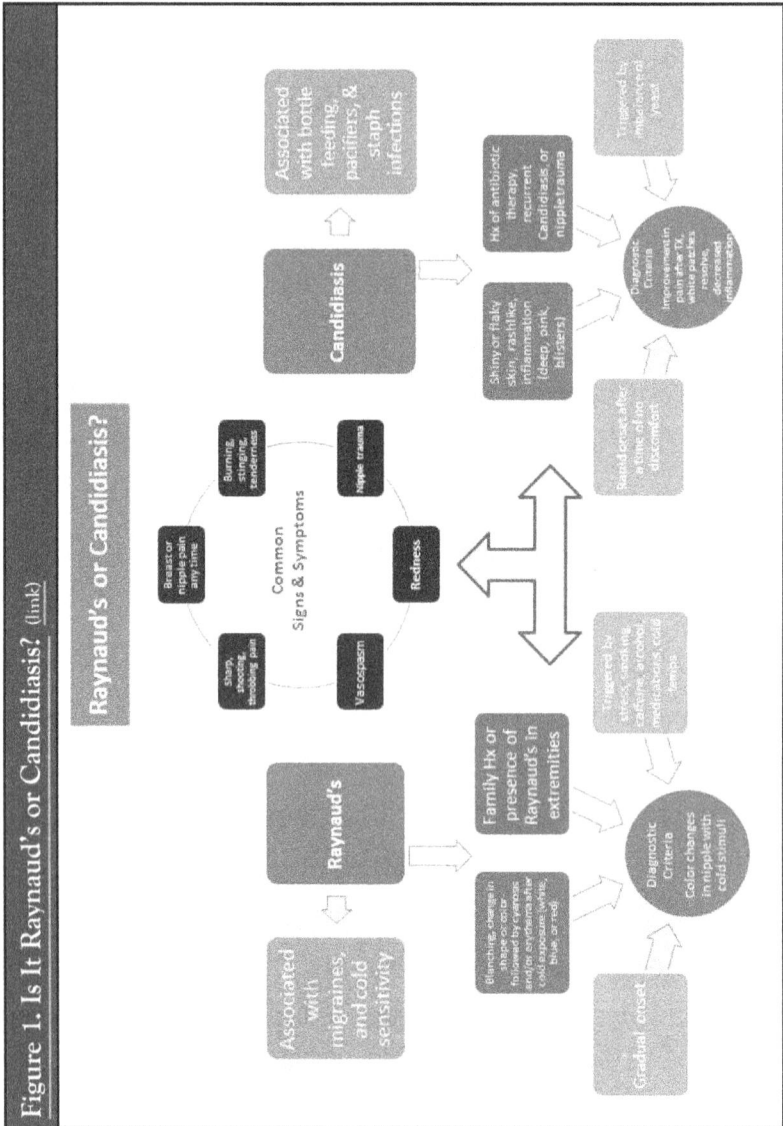

Figure 1. Is It Raynaud's or Candidiasis? (link)

This case study emphasizes the clinical dilemma faced by healthcare providers conducting an assessment for a patient presenting with breastfeeding and nipple pain. Our algorithm (Figure 1) presents the diagnostic criteria for these two complex conditions, with an emphasis on distinguishing characteristics. The intended purpose of an algorithm is to improve and standardize decisions while reducing error in situations of uncertainty. Use of this algorithm can help clinicians conduct a targeted breast assessment, identify distinguishing characteristics, and prevent unnecessary treatment.

Significance for Health Providers

Nurses and IBCLCs play an integral role as part of the healthcare team, providing evidence-based healthcare, advocating for resources, and identifying the need for referrals.

Breastfeeding education, care, and support from nurses as well as comprehensive lactation care including the management of complex breastfeeding problems from IBCLCs are standards of care for women and should be provided and accessible for the prevention, identification, and remediation of early breastfeeding challenges (Walker, 2008). Recommendation 5.6 of the Affordable Care Act ensures that breastfeeding counseling will be covered; but interpretation of who provides this counseling and for how long is unspecified (U.S. Department of Health & Human Services, 2012).

According to the *Surgeon General's Call to Action* (U.S. Department of Health & Human Services, 2011), new mothers need access to trained individuals with established relationships in the healthcare community who are flexible enough to meet mothers' needs outside of traditional work hours and locations, and who provide consistent information.

Yet evidenced-based knowledge, clinical skills, and attitudes of healthcare providers are known to be lacking, therefore creating barriers to breastfeeding women (Grossman et al., 2009). Educators are often forgotten as part of the healthcare team, but national organizations (United States Breastfeeding Committee, 2010; U.S. Department of Health & Human Services, 2011) are emphasizing the need for educators to be pivotal leaders in incorporating breastfeeding and human lactation education into all levels of curricula.

Additionally, this issue could be addressed through coordinated healthcare systems that partner with community networks in providing breastfeeding support so mothers have access to breastfeeding assistance after they return home. A model program is the Nurse and Family Partnership, an evidence-based home visiting program (http://www.nursefamilypartnership.org).

Raynaud's and Candidiasis can be challenging for clinicians to accurately assess and assist with evidence-based recommendations because they have similar clinical symptoms and a lack of standardized diagnostic tools.

This article offers an algorithm to help clinicians better distinguish between RP-n and Candidiasis based on the mother/infant dyad's history and physical examination. Medical treatment may be necessary for either condition, but non-pharmacological, as well as pharmacological measures should accompany those interventions.

Implications for Practice

The diagnosis of RP-n or Candidiasis does not mean breast-feeding must stop. However, more research needs to be conducted on better diagnostic tools, additional treatment options, and conditions/predisposing factors associated with both diseases.

Research is necessary to explain the pathogenesis of these conditions and to further educate clinicians on how to identify and assist with these two problems. Clinicians are cautioned to consider the differential diagnosis of nipple pain before recommending antifungal treatment.

References

Amir, L. H., Cullinane, M., Garland, S. M., Tabrizi, S. N., Donath, S. M., Bennett, C. M., Cooklin, A. R., Fisher, J., & Payne, M. S. (2011).The role of micro-organisms (*staphyloccus aureus and Candida albicans*) in the pathogenesis of breast pain and infection in lactating women: study protocol. *BMC Pregnancy and Childbirth, 11*, Retrieved from: http://www.biomedicalcentral. com/1471-2393/11/54

Anderson, J.E., Held, N., & Wright, K. (2004). Raynaud's phenomenon of the nipple: A treatable cause of painful breastfeeding. *Pediatrics, 113*, e360-e364.

Australian Breastfeeding Association. (2011). *Vasospasm*. Retreived from: https://breastfeeding.asn.au/bfinfo/vasospasm

Betzold, C. M. (2012). Results of microbial testing exploring the etiology of deep breast pain during lactation: A systematic review and meta-analysis of non-randomized trials. *Journal of Midwifery & Women's Health, 57*(4), 353-364.

Bonyata, K. (2011). *Nipple blanching and vasospasm*. KellyMom.com. Retrieved from: http://kellymom.com/bf/concerns/mom/nipple-blanching.html

Breastfeeding-problems.com. (2012). *Raynaud's Phenomenon*. Retrieved from http://www.breastfeeding-problems.com/Raynauds-phenomenon.html

Brent, N. (2001). Thrush in the breastfeeding dyad: Results of a survey on diagnosis and treatment. *Clinical Pediatrics, 40*, 503–506.

Delgado, S., Collado, M. C., Fernandez, L., & Rodriguez, J. M. (2009). Bacterial analysis of breast milk: A tool to differentiate Raynaud's phenomenon from infectious mastitis during lactation. *Current Microbiology, 59*, 59-64. doi:10.1007/s00284-009-9393-z

Garrison, C. P. (2002). Nipple vasospasms, Raynaud's syndrome, and nifedipine. *Journal of Human Lactation, 18*, 382-385. doi:10.1177/089033402237913

Goldfarb, L. (2002-2011). *Nipple vasospasm*. Breastfeeding Clinic, Herzl Family Practice Centre, SMBD Jewish General Hospital, Montreal, Quebec, Canada. Retrieved from: http://www.asklenore.com/breastfeeding/vasospasm.shtml

Grossman, X., Chauduri, J., Felman-Winter, L., Abrams, J., Niles Newton, K., Philipp, M., & Merewood, A. (2009). Hospital education in lactation practices (Project HELP): Does clinician education affect breastfeeding initiation and exclusivity in the hospital? *Birth, 36*, 54-59.

Hale, T. W., Bateman, T.L., Finkelman, M.A., & Berens, P. D. (2009). The absence of *Candida albicans* in milk samples of women with clinical symptoms of ductal candidiasis.*Breastfeeding Medicine, 4* (2), 57–61. doi: 10.1089/bfm.2008.0144

Hills, T. (2011). *Help for pregnant & breastfeeding moms*. The Raynaud's Association Blog Archive. Retrieved from: http://www.raynauds. org/2011/02/08/help-for-pregnant-breastfeeding-moms/

Hoen, O. L., & Backe, B. (2009). An underdiagnosed cause of nipple pain presented on a camera phone. *British Medical Journal, 339*. doi:10.1136/bmj.b2553

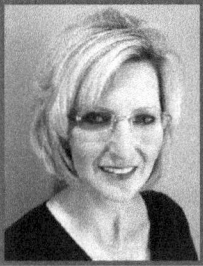

Genae D. Strong, PhD, CNM, RNC-OB, IBCLC, RLC, is an Assistant Professor at the University of Memphis, Loewenberg School of Nursing, with over 20 years of experience supporting breastfeeding women through teaching, research, and community service. Dr. Strong has published in the field of lactation and maintains a program of research focused on overcoming the barriers healthcare providers face while assisting the breastfeeding dyad. Currently, Dr. Strong is designing a breastfeeding educational curriculum for pre-licensure nursing students to improve their confidence, competence, and clinical experiences as recommended by national and international practice standards. Serving as the Memphis Area Lactation Consultant Association's (MALCA) president, and an active member of the Shelby County Breastfeeding Coalition (SCBC), Dr. Strong has a "strong" passion for improving the health of women and their infants.

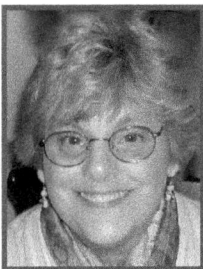

Nancy Mele, DSN, RN, is an Associate Professor at the University of Memphis Loewenberg School of Nursing. She has over 40 years of experience as a maternal child nurse and perinatal clinical specialist. Dr. Mele has worked with nursing mothers in the NICU, postpartum, and the community. She has taught prepared childbirth classes and formed a chapter of the La Leche League in the U.S., and while stationed overseas with her husband. Since entering academia, Dr. Mele has supported student learning through teaching about breastfeeding, serving women and children through the March of Dimes, and conducting research. She currently has two funded research studies on breastfeeding education for pre-licensure nursing students. Dr. Mele's doctoral education focused on health policy and she is currently active with several professional organizations in protecting women's and infant's health through legislative action. She is a curriculum and evaluation specialist and has plans to obtain her certification as a breastfeeding educator. Protecting and promoting health through breastfeeding has been her foundation for practice throughout her career.

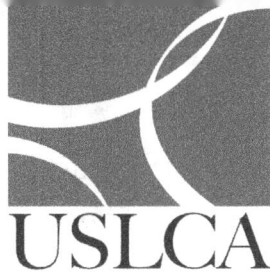

Are There Any Cures for Sore Nipples?

Marsha Walker, RN, IBCLC, RLC[1]

Keywords: Breastfeeding, sore nipples, treatments

Sore nipples are the bane of breastfeeding mothers. Nipple pain and/or damage ranks in the first 2 or 3 reasons for the early abandonment of breastfeeding. There exists a plethora of suggested remedies, many of which have little or no high-quality evidence to recommend their use. This article reviews approaches to managing sore nipples and suggests that more research be conducted to better remedy this ongoing problem.

Sore nipples are the bane of breastfeeding mothers. Some women experience nothing more than transient discomfort whereas others may suffer protracted, excruciating pain. Sore nipples are a common complaint of breastfeeding mothers and rank in the top two or three reasons why

1   Marshalact@gmail.com, Executive Director, National Alliance for Breastfeeding Advocacy

mothers terminate breastfeeding early in the lactation experience (Murimi, Dodge, Pope, & Erickson, 2010). This is especially true for African American and low-income mothers (Alexander, Dowling, & Furman, 2010). The incidence of sore nipples varies among studies, with as many as 96% of mothers reporting nipple discomfort at some point during the first 6 weeks postpartum (Ziemer, Paone, Schupay, & Cole, 1990).

Antenatal Interventions

For decades, mothers were taught antenatal nipple conditioning techniques in the hope of preventing sore nipples (see Box 1). Prenatal nipple conditioning techniques have, for the most part, been abandoned because high-quality evidence of their effectiveness is lacking.

Box 1. Historical Nipple Preparation Techniques
Nipple rolling
Rubbing with terry cloth towel
Hoffman's exercises (areolar stretching)
Avoidance of soap on nipples
Masse cream or other ointments
Air exposure under clothing
Breast shells
Nipple stretching

Researchers have measured the length of women's nipples prenatally and compared this to the LATCH (Jensen, Wallace, & Kelsay, 1994) score of their newborn infants. A prenatal nipple length of 7mm was considered the cut-off point for nipple length that facilitated successful latching. Mothers with a nipple length of less than 7mm had infants who more frequently scored less than 8 on the LATCH assessment tool. The 7mm nipple length might be a possible screening indicator that would signal the clinician to provide more intensive breastfeeding monitoring and support postpartum should a mother's nipple measure less than this (Puapornpong, Raungrongmorakot, Paritakul, Ketsuwam, & Wongin, 2013).

Some mothers with very flat or inverted nipples identified during the antenatal period, use a device called the Niplette to mechanically stretch the shortened internal tissues. The concept of tissue expansion through continuous long-term application of suction is derived from the plastic and aesthetic surgery disciplines. The Niplette is a transparent thimble-like mold with a syringe port through which the air is evacuated after placement over the nipple. The syringe is detached while the device is worn for eight or more hours during the day for the first 6 months of the pregnancy. A small amount of Vaseline or other lubricant is placed around the base of the mold to improve the seal.

Building on the concept of mechanical stretching, a product called the Supple Cup has been used for prenatal eversion of flat nipples (Bouchet-Horwitz, 2011). Supple

Cups are small thimble-like silicone cups that are squeezed to evacuate the air, placed over the nipple and released to create a vacuum that exerts traction on the nipple. They are worn under breast shells beginning at the 37th week of gestation.

Flat and Inverted Nipples

Dewey, Nommsen-Rivers, Heinig, and Cohen (2003) demonstrated that suboptimal breastfeeding behaviors were significantly associated with flat or inverted nipples.

Difficulty latching to the breast because of a nipple that cannot be elongated and placed properly in the infant's mouth can lead to not only sore nipples but also macerated/traumatized nipples that require more extensive interventions. Table 1 provides a summary of prenatal and postpartum interventions for flat or inverted nipples that may prevent or reduce pain and damage to nipples with these alterations.

There are many contributors to sore nipples, some of which include poor positioning, improper latch, dysfunctional or disorganized sucking, flat or inverted nipples, ankyloglossia, strong vacuum application by the infant (McClellan et al., 2008), C. albicans, eczema, Raynaud's phenomenon, vasospasm, nipple bleb, incorrect pump flange size, and bacterial infection. Interventions that address the source of the problem are the first line of action.

» Correction of positioning and latch is generally the first approach to eliminating sore nipples, with remediation often seen by the simple improvement of the infant's latch (Blair, Cadwell, Turner-Maffei,& Brimdyr, 2003; Darmangeat, 2011).

» Interventions are undertaken when sucking skills are compromised (Watson Genna, 2013).

Table 1. Summary of Interventions for Flat or Inverted Nipples		
Intervention	Pros	Cons
ANTENATAL		
Prenatal correction techniques	Familiarizes mothers with handling their breasts	Is generally ineffective and is seldom recommended
Prenatal mechanical stretching with Niplette	Is an effective tissue expander	Has the potential for pain and bleeding if too much suction is applied
Prenatal mechanical stretching with Supple Cup	Gradually everts nipples	May experience some discomfort and/or scant bleeding
Prenatal surgical correction	Is very effective in correcting inverted nipples	Has a high potential for severing ducts within the nipple and impeding breastfeeding; generally not recommended
POSTBIRTH		
Cold compress prior to feeding	Will cause contraction of erector muscles	May not be sufficient to affect an inverted nipple or provide enough graspable tissue for some infants
Pull and roll nipple prior to feeding	Is a fast and easy method to evert a nipple	May not stay everted long enough for some infants or provide sufficient graspable tissue
Pop out nipple prior to feeding by fingertip pressure behind the nipple	Is a fast and easy method to evert a nipple	May not be effective with inverted nipples or nipples tightly tethered to underlying tissue
Breast pump	Extends nipple away from areola, stretching it into nipple tunnel	Distributes vacuum over a large area; causes nipple swelling; nipples may not stay everted very long
A 10-ml modified syringe used prior to each feeding (Kesaree, Banapurmath, Banapurmath, & Shamanur, 1993)	Is easy, inexpensive, effective method to evert nipple	May not be allowed by some hospitals that restrict the use of non-FDA approved devices
Evert-It Nipple Enhancer	Is an FDA approved device for everting flat nipples	Have little data about its effectiveness
Latch Assist	Is an FDA approved device for everting flat nipples	Have little data about its effectiveness
Supple Cups	Can be worn in between or just prior to feedings	There is only one small study demonstrating their effectiveness
Breast shells	May help reduce areolar edema surrounding nipple	May cause tissue damage if areolar edema is present and shells are worn for extended periods
Reverse pressure softening (Cotterman, 2004)	Helps reveal nipple enveloped by edematous areola	May not expose enough of the nipple for infant to grasp
Teacup hold	May provide sufficient tissue for a good latch	Is not effective on an engorged breast or edematous areola
Dimple ring	Is a simple device to hold open a dimpled nipple for air drying	May be difficult to locate
Nipple shield	Is useful if no other techniques or devices are effective in facilitating a good latch	May be difficult for some infants to learn to latch without the shield
Niplette	Is effective in stretching the nipple	Loses suction if milk gets into the mold

Source: Walker, M. (2010). *The nipple and areola in breastfeeding and lactation.* Amarillo, TX: Hale Publishing.

» Ankyloglossia (tongue-tie) is generally improved by frenotomy (Buryk, Bloom, & Shope, 2011; Dollberg, Botzer, Grunis, & Mimouni, 2006).

» *C. albicans* should be identified and treated either topically and/or systemically (Morrill, Heinig, Pappagianis, & Dewey, 2004; Panjaitan, Amir, Costs, Rudland, & Tabrizi, 2008; Porter & Schach, 2004).

» Eczema usually responds to removal of an irritant or allergen and/or the application of topical corticosteroids (Amir, 1993; Barankin & Gross,2004).

» Raynaud's phenomenon may respond to the application of warmth and avoidance of cold exposure, the discontinuation of vasoconstricting drugs, such as caffeine and nicotine, and/or the use of nifedipine (Anderson, Held, & Wright, 2004; Lawlor-Smith & Lawlor-Smith, 1996; O'Sullivan & Keith, 2011; Wu, Chason, & Wong, 2012).

» In a study by O'Hara (2012), nipple bleb histology showed the lack of bacteria or fungi and the presence of immune cells when the rubbery white nipple pore blockages were removed and studied microscopically. Blebs resistant to conventional treatments were removed by O'Hara using a punch biopsy tool that resolved the pain and symptoms. The presence of immune cells indicated a tissue reaction to milk that had leaked from the nipple pore and infiltrated into the surrounding tissue. Based on these findings,

O'Hara recommended a short daily course of a very thin layer of a mid-potency steroid under an occlusive dressing to enhance penetration of the steroid into the inflamed and fibrotic tissue. Nipple blebs appeared to be an inflammatory response to nipple trauma in some women.

» An incorrect pump flange size has been identified as a source of nipple pain for some mothers expressing their milk. Nipples swell during pumping (Wilson-Clay & Hoover, 2008) and some mothers may require a larger flange size to prevent or remain free of pain (Meier, Motyhowski, & Zuleger, 2004). Some mothers may even need a different size flange for each breast, or that as lactation progresses they may actually require a smaller shield (Jones & Hilton, 2009). If mothers cannot achieve a comfortable fit by changing flange sizes, they may find relief by using a product called Pumpin Pal. This is an angled flange that may better accommodate some breasts (Walker, 2010).

» Once the integrity of the nipple skin has been breached, it becomes highly susceptible to colonization and infection by bacteria, such as *S. aureus*. This can lead to prolonged nipple pain, delayed healing, complications, and the need for more aggressive interventions (see Box 2).

There is an association between severe nipple soreness and colonization and infection of the nipple by *S. aureus*, so careful washing of the nipple with soap and water and the application of mupirocin 2% ointment (Bactroban) may be effective in the early stages of the infection (Livingstone, Willis, & Berkowitz, 1996).

Bacteria can grow in colonies and protect the colony with a shield or coating called a biofilm. These biofilms protect the bacteria from antibiotic therapy and the mother's immune system. To disrupt this protective

---

Box 2. Potential Sequelae of Cracked Nipples

- S. *aureus* as a resident bacteria on the nipple skin.

- Nipple trauma and cracks breech nipple skin integrity.

- S. *aureus* strains penetrate superficial layers of broken epidermis.

- Toxins produced cause inflammation, epidermal separation, and blisters.

- Blisters open causing erosions that become covered by a yellow, crusted exudate.

- Pain occurs that could be sufficient to inhibit letdown or reduce milk transfer leading to milk stasis.

- Infection might occur in ascending lactiferous ducts.

- Mastitis could develop if infection is not treated.

- Abscess may develop if mastitis is not treated.

Source: Walker, M. (2010). *The nipple and areola in breastfeeding and lactation.* Amarillo, TX: Hale Publishing.

biofilm, the nipple wound should be washed with soap and water once a day, followed by a coating of mupirocin. Once the biofilm has been disrupted or broken down, the topical antibiotic can reach the affected area, promote wound healing, and prevent progression to a florid infection (Ryan, 2007).

Much of a mother's nipple pain may stem from inflammation. Low- to medium-strength steroids applied as a thin coat to the nipples might provide pain relief (Huggins & Billon, 1993). If clinicians see exudate from the nipple wound, if erythema (redness) increases, or dry scabs do not form, then systemic antibiotics may be necessary. If the painful nipples persist, this could be a combination of yeast and bacterial infection, in which case clinicians may wish to use miconazole 2% as the antifungal preparation, along with mupirocin and a topical steroid (Porter & Schach, 2004). Eglash and Proctor (2007) reported on a set of signs and symptoms (nipple cracks that did not heal despite systemic antibiotics, dull throbbing of the breasts, sharp shooting pains, breast pain on palpation), whose laboratory findings of the cultured milk were typical of infections caused by small colony variants (SCVs) of *staphylococci*. SVCs cause persistent, antibiotic-resistant, refractory infections that can take many weeks of antibiotics to clear (von Eiff, Peters, & Becker, 2006). Treatment options for cracked or damaged nipples appear in Box 3.

No matter what the cause of sore nipples, mothers and clinicians often want an additional treatment that will reduce the pain and hasten the healing of traumatized

Box 3. Treatment Options for Cracked or Damaged Nipples

Correct positioning and latch.

If there is a break in the nipple skin:

Wash nipple with soap and water once each day.

Apply topical mupirocin.

Avoid pacifier use or wash pacifiers thoroughly with soap and water.

Apply topical low strength steroids for inflammation.

If exudate is seen, erythema increases, or dry scab is absent:

Add systemic antibiotics.

If C. *albicans* is suspected, add topical 2% miconazole.

If infection is recurrent or persistent:

Treat infant with nasal mupirocin because the infant may be a carrier of S. *aureus* and infect or reinfect the mother's nipple (Amir, Garland, & Lumley, 2006).

Test for SCV; ask for culture and sensitivity laboratory testing.

If SCV are present, switch to macrolide therapy.

Be watchful for an ascending infection (mastitis).

Correct anemia.

Source: Walker, M. (2010). *The nipple and areola in breastfeeding and lactation.* Amarillo, TX: Hale Publishing.

tissue. Remedies for sore nipples have been seen in the medical literature since the 17th century, with all manners of plasters, poultices, and ointments applied topically as comfort measures.

In spite of the plethora of treatments for sore nipples that have been recommended over the years (Table 2), no single treatment agent has been shown to be clearly superior to all others (Morland- Schultz & Hill, 2005).

Research studies on sore nipple interventions use differing methodologies, are inconclusive, and often inconsistent or contradictory in outcomes.

When comparing treatments, some agents yield better results than others (see Table 3). Recommendations for sore-nipple therapies do not always have high-level research to support their use or may extrapolate approaches used in other disciplines. Plant extracts are often the base of topical wound treatments because many produce flavonoid compounds with phenolic components. These phytochemicals are highly reactive and act to neutralize the effects of free radicals or initiate biological effects.

Green Tea Bags

Green tea includes a class of polyphenol compounds, called catechins, that enhance natural wound healing (Hsu, 2005).

At certain concentrations, green tea polyphenols have the ability to stimulate aged keratinocytes (epidermal cells that synthesize keratin—the cornified [horny] layer of skin

Table 2. Some Treatments for Sore Nipples Over the Years

Warm-water compresses	Lanolin	Saline soaks
Wet tea bags	Vitamin E oil	Hydrogel dressings
Triple antibiotic	Herbal and botanical preparations	Olive oil
All-purpose nipple ointment	Homeopathic preparations	Peppermint water
Peppermint gel	Commercial nipple creams	Expressed breast milk
Virgin coconut oil	A & D ointment	Lotrimin AF
LED phototherapy	Bacitracin	Bactroban
Micatin	Monistat	Medihoney
Systemic antibiotics	Gentian violet	Nifedipine
Soft-laser therapy	Systemic antibiotics	Topical lecithin

Note. LED = light-emitting diode.

Table 3. Comparison of Topical Agents for Treatment or Prevention of Nipple Pain			
Agent	Positive Results	Equivalent Results	Negative Results
Expressed mother's milk (EMM)	Superior to lanolin (Mohammadzadeh, Farhat, & Esmaeily, 2005)	Equivalent to lanolin (Hewat & Ellis, 1987)	Inferior to warm-water compresses (Buchko et al, 1994; Pugh et al., 1996) Inferior to keeping nipples dry and clean (Akkuzu & Taskin, 2000) Inferior to lanolin (Coca & Abrao, 2008) Inferior to peppermint water (Sayyah et al., 2007) Inferior to lanolin (Abou-Dakn, Fluhr, Gensch, & Wockel, 2011)
Tea bag compress		Equivalent to lanolin in neither preventing nor reducing soreness (Riordan, 1985) Equivalent to warm-water compress (Lavergne, 1997)	Inferior to warm-water compresses (Buchko et al., 1994)
Warm-water compress	Superior to tea bags or EMM (Buchko et al., 1994) Superior to lanolin and EMM (Pugh et al., 1996)	Equivalent to tea bags (Lavergne, 1997)	Inferior to keeping nipples dry and clean (Akkuzu & Taskin, 2000)
Lanolin	Superior to no treatment after 5 days (Spangler & Hildebrandt, 1993) Superior to EMM (Coca & Abrao, 2008) Superior to EMM (Abou-Dakn et al., 2011)	Equivalent to EMM (Hewat & Ellis, 1987) Equivalent to tea bags in neither preventing nor reducing soreness (Riordan, 1985) Not more effective than all-purpose nipple ointment in healing sore nipples (Dennis, Schottle, Hodnett, & McQueen, 2012)	Inferior to warm water compresses (Pugh et al., 1996) Inferior to hydrogel dressings (Dodd & Chalmers, 2003) Inferior to EMM (Mohammadzadeh et al., 2005) Inferior to peppermint gel (Melli et al, 2007)
Hydrogel dressing	Superior to lanolin (Dodd & Chalmers, 2003)		
Peppermint gel	Superior to lanolin (Melli et al., 2007)		
Peppermint water	Superior to EMM (Sayyah et al, 2007)		
All-purpose nipple ointment		Not more effective than lanolin in healing sore nipples (Dennis et al., 2012)	
LED phototherapy	Superior to standard treatment of proper positioning and latch, frequency and length of feedings, and general breastfeeding education (Chaves, Araújo, Santos, Pinotti, & Oliveira, 2012)		

Note. LED = light-emitting diode.
Source: Lochner, J. E., Livingston, C. J., & Judkins, D. Z. (2009). Clinical inquiries: Which interventions are best for alleviating nipple pain in nursing mothers? *Journal of Family Practice, 58*(11), 612a–612c.

that is a protective layer to mechanical injury, microbial invasion, and water loss) and reduce healing time of epidermal wounds (Hsu et al., 2003). Mothers may find some relief from abraded, sore nipples by the use of green tea bags soaked in warm water.

Peppermint

Peppermint (*Mentha piperita*) has been shown to have a calming and numbing effect on skin irritations (Blumenthal, Goldberg, & Brinckmann, 2000); increase tissue flexibility and improve its resistance to cracking (Schelz, Molnar, & Hohmann, 2006); demonstrate strong antibacterial and anti-inflammatory activity; and possess both fungistatic and fungicidal activities (Mimica-Dukic & Boz˘in, 2008; Mimica-Dukic´, Boz˘in, Sokovic´, Mihajlovic´, & Matavulj, 2003).

In a study on the prophylactic use of peppermint gel on nipples, mothers in three groups were instructed to either rub peppermint gel on their nipples following each feeding, rub lanolin on their nipples after feedings, or use a placebo following feedings. The rate of cracked nipples was 22.6% in the placebo group, 6.9% in the lanolin group, and 3.8% in the peppermint gel group (Melli et al., 2007). Although the use of peppermint gel was more effective on the prevention of cracked nipples, Sayyah and colleagues (2007) found that even peppermint water used prophylactically on nipples was three times more effective in preventing nipple cracks than expressed breast milk (27% expressed breast milk compare with 9%peppermint water).

Olive Oil

Hydrophilic phenols are the most abundant antioxidants in virgin olive oil with both antioxidant and anti-inflammatory attributes.

Olive oil contains significant amounts of *squalene*, the main component of skin surface polyunsaturated lipids. As an emollient, squalene is easily absorbed deep into the skin helping to restore suppleness and flexibility (two positive attributes of nipple skin that helps resist cracking and damage).

Ozonated olive oil was effective in animal models for accelerating wound repair (Kim et al., 2009; Sakazaki et al., 2007). Olive oil is treated with gaseous ozone to produce a product to which bacteria cannot mount resistance. Ozonated olive oil possesses a wide range of activities that operate during all phases of the wound healing process. Ozonated olive oil is available commercially, but no studies have been found that discussed using the preparation for healing damaged nipples.

Virgin Coconut Oil

Virgin coconut oil has long been used in tropical countries, and Ayurvedic medicine for skin disorders and wound healing. Lactation consultants have anecdotally reported positive outcomes on sore nipples from the use of virgin coconut oil, but no studies could be located that used virgin coconut oil on sore or damaged nipples. In an animal study, Nevin and Rajamohan (2010) found that wounds treated with virgin coconut oil healed much faster than untreated wounds, most likely because of the variety of biologically active ingredients in coconut oil that serve to hasten steps in the wound healing process. Virgin coconut oil was found to be superior to olive oil in a study that compared their ability to eliminate *S. aureus* from adult skin with atopic dermatitis. Virgin coconut oil demonstrated broad spectrum activity against *S. aureus,* fungi, and viruses (Verallo-Rowell, Dillaque, & Syah-Tjundawan, 2008).

Honey

Honey has been shown to have wound healing and antibacterial properties (Moore et al., 2001), but seems dependent on the type of honey, geographical location, and flower from which the final product is derived.

Medical-grade honey (Medihoney) is an effective would healing agent and antibacterial preparation (Robson, Dodd, & Thomas, 2009). Merckoll, Jonassen, Vad, Jeansson, and Melby (2009) reported that Medihoney was bactericidal against multiple species of bacteria, including *methicillin resistant Staphylococcus aureus* (MRSA). Medihoney is effective against antibiotic resistant organisms, with a low likelihood of bacteria becoming resistant to it. Furthermore, Medihoney has the ability to penetrate biofilms, a property that is important in infected wounds that are not healing (Merckoll et al., 2009). Medihoney is treated to eliminate botulism spores, and has been used anecdotally by many clinicians to help heal damaged nipples.

Warm-Water Compresses

Simple warm-water compresses promote comfort, enhance blood flow to wounded tissues, and aid in the removal of cellular waste products. Mothers can add one-fourth to one-half teaspoon of salt per quart of warm water and apply the saline soak for 10 min.

Commercial Nipple Creams

Commercial nipple creams contain multiple ingredients, not all of which have been shown to be safe or effective. The Food and Drug Administration (FDA) issued a warning in 2008 regarding the potential hazards of using a certain nipple cream because of the potential harm its ingredients could cause to both mother and infant.

Numerous other preparations are used on sore or traumatized nipples, with many having little evidence for their safety and effectiveness.

A sample intervention plan for sore nipples appears in Box 4. Although mothers may be able to achieve normal milk production in the face of experiencing sore nipples (McClellen, Hepworth, Kent et al., 2012), nipple pain (even without visible trauma) negatively interferes not only with breastfeeding itself, but also with a mother's mood, general activity, and sleep (McClellan, Hepworth, Garbin et al., 2012). Additional research is essential for providing high-quality evidence to delineate the best options in treating sore and damaged nipples.

Box 4. Sample Intervention Plans for Sore Nipples

Preventive Strategies

- Use optimal positioning. Assess latch, suck, and swallowing and correct positioning if necessary.

- Use a modified syringe, nipple rolling, or tea cup hold to assist with latch if nipples are flat.

- Check to make sure the infant's mouth is open to 160° angle, with lips flared outward, and neck slightly extended.

- If pumping, assure the flange is large enough to prevent nipple strangulation in the flange's tunnel.

- Provide relief from engorgement.

- Avoid pacifiers until breastfeeding is well established.

- Correct ankyloglossia if present.

- Apply peppermint water or peppermint gel to nipples after each early feeding.

When Nipples Are Already Sore

In addition to the aforementioned measures, the following preparations may be tried for soothing, pain relief, and healing:

Warm-water compresses

Warm green tea bag compresses

Peppermint water or gel

Olive oil

Coconut oil

Medihoney

Hydrogel dressing

Nipple shield, if nothing else is working and the mother verbalizes her desire to stop breastfeeding

Source: Walker, M. (2010). *The nipple and areola in breastfeeding and lactation.* Amarillo, TX: Hale Publishing.

Hydrogel Dressings

Hydrogel dressings for healing sore, traumatized, or macerated nipples is a therapy adapted from wound healing interventions on other parts of the body. These dressings are water based and often a combination of water and glycerin in a polymer matrix. Their value lies in their ability to maintain moisture, inhibit scab or crust formation, reduce pain, and enhance epithelial migration for wound repair.

Researchers have noted that mothers frequently find significant relief from pain when using hydrogel dressings between feedings (Cable, Stewart, & Davis, 1997; Dodd & Chalmers, 2003; Cadwell, Turner-Maffei, Blair, Brimdyr, & McInerney, 2004).

Hydrogel dressings may be a possible option in the treatment of nipples with open sores or cracks with exudate. The dressing absorbs wound discharge and prevents the nipple skin from adhering to the mother's bra. Clinicians should choose a hydrogel dressing that does not require adhesives to stick to the breast, as some mothers have complained that hydrogel dressings with adhesive backings irritate the skin when removed.

When the dressing is removed for a feeding, there should be no residue or small pieces of the dressing that adhere to the nipples. Mothers may also find additional relief from pain by chilling the hydrogel dressing in the refrigerator prior to application.

References

Abou-Dakn, M., Fluhr, J. W., Gensch, M., & Wockel, A. (2011). Positive effect of HPA lanolin versus expressed breastmilk on painful and damaged nipples during lactation. *Skin Pharmacologyand Physiology, 24*, 27–35.

Akkuzu, G., & Taskin, L. (2000). Impacts of breast-care techniques on prevention of possible postpartum nipple problems. *Professional Care of Mother and Child, 10*, 38–41.

Alexander, A., Dowling, D., & Furman, L. (2010). What do pregnant low-income women say about breastfeeding? *Breastfeeding Medicine, 5*, 17–23.

Amir, L. (1993). Eczema of the nipple and breast: A case report. *Journal of Human Lactation, 9*, 173–175.

Amir, L. H., Garland, S. M., & Lumley, J. (2006). A case-control study of mastitis: Nasal carriage of *Staphylococcus aureus*. BMC *Family Practice, 7*, 57.

Anderson, J. E., Held, N., & Wright, K. (2004). Raynaud's phenomenon of the nipple: A treatable cause of painful breastfeeding. *Pediatrics, 113*, e360–e364.

Barankin, B., & Gross, M. S. (2004). Nipple and areolar eczema in the breastfeeding woman. *Journal of Cutaneous Medicine and Surgery, 8*, 126–130.

Blair, A., Cadwell, K., Turner-Maffei, C., & Brimdyr, K. (2003). The relationship between positioning, the breastfeeding dynamic, the latching process and pain in breastfeeding mothers with sore nipples. *Breastfeeding Review, 11*, 5–10.

Blumenthal, M., Goldberg, A., & Brinckmann, J. (2000). *Herbal medicine: Expanded Commission E Monographs*. Newton, MA: Integrative Medicine Communications.

Bouchet-Horwitz, J. (2011). The use of Supple Cups for flat, retracting, and inverted nipples. *Clinical Lactation, 2*(3), 30–33.

Buchko, B. L., Pugh, L. C., Bishop, B. A., Cochran, J. F., Smith, L. R., & Lerew, D. J. (1994). Comfort measures in breastfeeding, primiparous women. *Journal of Obstetric, Gynecologic and Neonatal Nursing, 23*, 46–52.

Buryk, M., Bloom, D., & Shope, T. (2011). Efficacy of neonatal release of ankyloglossia: A randomized trial. *Pediatrics, 128*, 280–288.

Cable, B., Stewart, M., & Davis, J. (1997). Nipple wound care: A new approach to an old problem. *Journal of Human Lactation, 13*, 313–318.

Cadwell, K., Turner-Maffei, C., Blair, A., Brimdyr, K., & McInerney, Z. (2004). Pain reduction and treatment of sore nipples in nursing mothers. *Journal of Perinatal Education, 13*, 29–35.

Chaves, M. E., Araújo, A. R., Santos, S. F., Pinotti, M., & Oliveira, L. S. (2012). LED phototherapy improves healing of nipple trauma: A pilot study. *Photomedicine and Laser Surgery, 30*, 172–178.

Coca, K. P., & Abrao, A. C. F. V. (2008). An evaluation of the effect of lanolin in healing nipple injuries. *Acta Paulista de Enfermagem, 21*, 11–16.

Cotterman, K. J. (2004). Reverse pressure softening: A simple tool to prepare areola for easier latching during engorgement. *Journal of Human Lactation, 20*, 227–237.

Darmangeat, V. (2011). The frequency and resolution of nipple pain when latch is improved in a private practice. *Clinical Lactation, 2*(3), 22–24.

Dennis, C.-L., Schottle, N., Hodnett, E., & McQueen, K. (2012). An all-purpose nipple ointment versus lanolin in treating painful damaged nipples in breastfeeding women: A randomized controlled trial. *Breastfeeding Medicine, 7*(6), 473–479. http://dx.doi.org/10.1089/bfm.2011.0121

Dewey, K. G., Nommsen-Rivers, L., Heinig, M. J., & Cohen, R.J. (2003). Risk factors for suboptimal infant breastfeeding behavior, delayed onset of lactation, and excess neonatal weight loss. *Pediatrics, 112*, 607–619.

Dodd, V., & Chalmers, C. (2003). Comparing the use of hydrogel dressings to lanolin ointment with lactating mothers. *Journal of Obstetric, Gynecologic, and Neonatal Nursing, 32*, 486–494.

Dollberg, S., Botzer, E., Grunis, E., & Mimouni, F. B. (2006). Immediate nipple pain relief after frenotomy in breastfed infants with ankyloglossia: A randomized, prospective study. *Journal of Pediatric Surgery, 41*, 1598–1600.

Eglash, A., & Proctor, R. (2007). A breastfeeding mother with chronic breast pain. *Breastfeeding Medicine, 2*, 99–103.

Food and Drug Administration. (2008). *FDA warns consumers against using Mommy's Bliss nipple cream: Product can be harmful to nursing infants.* Retrieved from http://www.fda.gov/NewsEvents/Newsroom/PressAnnouncements/2008/ucm116900.htm

Hewat, R. J., & Ellis, D. J. (1987). A comparison of the effectiveness of two methods of nipple care. *Birth, 14*, 41–45.

Hsu, S. (2005). Green tea and the skin. *Journal of the American Academy of Dermatology, 52*, 1049–1059.

Hsu, S., Bollag, W. B., Lewis, J., Huang, Q., Singh, B., Sharawy, M., . . . Schuster, G. (2003). Green tea polyphenols induce differentiation and proliferation in epidermal keratinocytes. *Journal of Pharmacology and Experimental Therapeutics, 306,* 29–34.

Huggins, K. E., & Billon, S. F. (1993). Twenty cases of persistent sore nipples: Collaboration between lactation consultant and dermatologist. *Journal of Human Lactation, 9,* 155–160.

Jensen D., Wallace S., & Kelsay, P. (1994). LATCH: a breastfeeding charting system and documentation tool. *Journal of Obstetric, Gynecologic and Neonatal Nursing, 23,* 27–32.

Jones, E., & Hilton, S. (2009). Correctly fitting breast shields are the key to lactation success for pump dependent mothers following preterm delivery. *Journal of Neonatal Nursing, 15,* 14–17.

Kesaree, N., Banapurmath, C. R., Banapurmath, S., & Shamanur, K. (1993). Treatment of inverted nipples using a disposable syringe. *Journal of Human Lactation, 9,* 27–29.

Kim, H. S., Noh, S. U., Han, Y. W., Kim, K. M., Kang, H., Kim, H. O., & Park, Y. M. (2009). Therapeutic effects of topical application of ozone on acute cutaneous wound healing. *Journal of Korean Medical Science, 24,* 368–374.

Lavergne, N. A. (1997). Does application of tea bags to sore nipples while breastfeeding provide effective relief? *Journal of Obstetric, Gynecologic, and Neonatal Nursing, 26,* 53–58.

Lawlor-Smith, L., & Lawlor-Smith, C. (1996). Nipple vasospasm in the breastfeeding woman. *Breastfeeding Review, 4,* 37–39.

Livingstone, V. H., Willis, C. E., & Berkowitz, J. (1996). Staphylococcus aureus and sore nipples. *Canadian Family Physician, 42,* 654–659.

Lochner, J. E., Livingston, C. J., & Judkins, D. Z. (2009). Clinical inquiries: Which interventions are best for alleviating nipple pain in nursing mothers? *Journal of Family Practice, 58*(11), 612a–612c.

McClellan, H., Geddes, D., Kent, J., Garbin, C., Mitoulas, L., & Hartmann, P. (2008). Infants of mothers with persistent nipple pain exert strong sucking vacuums. *Acta Paediatrica, 97,* 1205–1209.

McClellen, H. L., Hepworth, A. R., Garbin, C. P., Rowan, M. K., Deacon, J., Hartmann, P. E., & Geddes, D. T. (2012). Nipple pain during breastfeeding with or without visible trauma. *Journal of Human Lactation, 28,* 511–521.

McClellen, H. L., Hepworth, A. R., Kent, J. C., Garbin, C. P., Williams, T. M., Hartmann, P. E., & Geddes, D. T. (2012).

Breastfeeding frequency, milk volume, and duration in motherinfant dyads with persistent nipple pain. *Breastfeeding Medicine, 7*, 275–281.

Meier, P., Motyhowski, J., & Zuleger, J. (2004). Choosing a correctly fitted breast shield for milk expression. *Medela Messenger, 21*, 8–9.

Melli, M. S., Rashidi, M. R., Nokhoodchi, A., Tagavi, S., Farzadi, L., Sadaghat, K., . . . Sheshvan, M. K. (2007). A randomized trial of peppermint gel, lanolin ointment, and placebo gel to prevent nipple crack in primiparous breastfeeding women. *Medical Science Monitor, 13*, CR406–CR411.

Merckoll, P., Jonassen, T. O., Vad, M. E., Jeansson, S. L., & Melby, K. K. (2009). Bacteria, biofilm and honey: A study of the effects of honey on 'planktonic' and biofilm-embedded wound bacteria. *Scandinavian Journal of Infectious Diseases, 41*, 341–347.

Mimica-Dukic´, N., & Bozˇin, B. (2008). Mentha L. species (Lamiaceae) as promising sources of bioactive secondary metabolites. *Current Pharmaceutical Design, 14*, 3141–3150.

Mimica-Dukic´, N., Bozˇin, B., Sokovic´, M., Mihajlovic´, B., & Matavulj, M. (2003). Antimicrobial and antioxidant activities of three Mentha species essential oils. *Planta Medica, 69*, 413–419.

Mohammadzadeh, A., Farhat, A., & Esmaeily, H. (2005). The effect of breast milk and lanolin on sore nipples. *Saudi Medical Journal, 26*, 1231–1234.

Moore, O. A., Smith, L. A., Campbell, F., Seers, K., McQuay, H. J., & Moore, R. A. (2001). *BMC Complementary and Alternative Medicine, 1*, 2.

Morland-Schultz, K., & Hill, P. D. (2005). Prevention of and therapies for nipple pain: A systematic review. *Journal of Obstetric, Gynecologic, and Neonatal Nursing, 34*, 428–437.

Morrill, J. F., Heinig, M. J., Pappagianis, D., & Dewey, K. G. (2004). Diagnostic value of signs and symptoms of mammary candidosis among lactating women. *Journal of Human Lactation, 20*, 288–295.

Murimi, M., Dodge, C. M., Pope, J., & Erickson, D. (2010). Factors that influence breastfeeding decisions among Special Supplemental Nutrition Program for Women, Infants, and Children participants from central Louisiana. *Journal of the American Dietetic Association, 110*, 624–627.

Nevin, K. G., & Rajamohan, T. (2010). Effect of topical application of virgin coconut oil on skin components and antioxidant status during dermal wound healing in young rats. *Skin Pharmacology and Physiology, 23*, 290–297.

O'Hara, M. A. (2012). Bleb histology reveals inflammatory infiltrate that regresses with topical steroids: A case series. *Breastfeeding Medicine, 7*(Suppl 1), S-2.

O'Sullivan, S., & Keith, M. P. (2011). Raynaud phenomenon of the nipple: A rare finding in rheumatology clinic. *Journal of Clinical Rheumatology, 17,* 371–372.

Panjaitan, M., Amir, L. H., Costs, A.-M., Rudland, E., & Tabrizi, S. (2008). Polymerase chain reaction in detection of *Candida albicans* for confirmation of clinical diagnosis of nipple thrush. *Breastfeeding Medicine, 3,* 185–187.

Porter, J., & Schach, B. (2004). Treating sore, possibly infected nipples. *Journal of Human Lactation, 20,* 221–222.

Puapornpong, P., Raungrongmorakot, K., Paritakul, P., Ketsuwam, S., & Wongin, S. (2013). Nipple length and its relation to success in breastfeeding. *Journal of the Medical Association of Thailand, 96*(Suppl. 1), S1–S4.

Pugh, L. C., Buchko, B. L., Bishop, B. A., Cochran, J. F., Smith, L. R., & Lerew, D. J. (1996). A comparison of topical agents to relieve nipple pain and enhance breastfeeding. *Birth, 23,* 88–93.

Riordan, J. (1985). The effectiveness of topical agents in reducing nipple soreness of breastfeeding mothers. *Journal of Human Lactation, 1,* 36–41.

Robson, V., Dodd, S., & Thomas, S. (2009). Standardized antibacterial honey (Medihoney) with standard therapy in wound care: Randomized clinical trial. *Journal of Advanced Nursing, 65,* 565–575.

Ryan, T. J. (2007). Infection following soft tissue injury: Its role in wound healing. *Current Opinion in Infectious Disease, 20,* 124–128..

Sakazaki, F., Kataoka, H., Okuno, T., Ueno, H., Semma, M., Ichikawa, A., & Nakamuro, K. (2007). Ozonated olive oil enhances the growth of granulation tissue in a mouse model of pressure ulcer. *Ozone: Science & Engineering, 29,* 503–507.

Sayyah, M. M., Rashidi, M. R., Delazar, A., Madarek, E., Kargar Maher, M. H., Ghasemzadeh, A., . . . Tahmasebi, Z. (2007). Effect of peppermint water on prevention of nipple cracks in lactating primiparous women: A randomized controlled trial. *International Breastfeeding Journal, 2,* 7.

Schelz, Z., Molnar, J., & Hohmann, J. (2006). Antimicrobial and antiplasmid activities of essential oils. *Fitoterapia, 77,* 279–285.

Spangler, A., & Hildebrandt, E. (1993). The effect of modified lanolin on nipple pain/damage during the first ten days of breastfeeding. *International Journal of Childbirth Education, 8,* 15–19.

Verallo-Rowell, V. M., Dillaque, K. M., & Syah-Tjundawan, B. S. (2008). Novel antibacterial and emollient effects of coconut and virgin olive oils in adult atopic dermatitis. *Dermatitis, 19,* 308–315.

von Eiff, C., Peters, G., & Becker, K. (2006). The small colony variant (SCV) concept—The role of staphylococcal SCVs in persistent infections. *Injury, 37,* S26–S33.

Walker, M. (2010). *The nipple and areola in breastfeeding and lactation.* Amarillo, TX: Hale Publishing.

Watson Genna, C. (2013). *Supporting sucking skills in breastfeeding infants.* Burlington, MA: Jones & Bartlett Learning.

Wilson-Clay, B., & Hoover, K. (2008). *The breastfeeding atlas* (4th ed.). Austin, TX: LactNews Press.

Wu, M., Chason, R., & Wong, M. (2012). Raynaud's phenomenon of the nipple. *Obstetrics and Gynecology, 119,* 447–449.

Ziemer, M. M., Paone, J. P., Schupay, J., & Cole, E. (1990). Methods to prevent and manage nipple pain in breastfeeding women. *Western Journal of Nursing Research, 12,* 732–744.

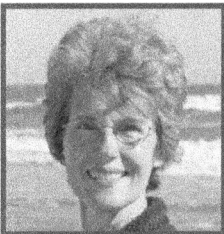

Marsha Walker, RN, IBCLC, RLC, is a registered nurse, lactation consultant, and breastfeeding advocate at the state and federal levels. She is the executive director of the National Alliance for Breastfeeding Advocacy (NABA), the IBFAN organization that monitors the International Code of Marketing of Breastmilk Substitutes in the United States. Marsha is NABA's representative to the US Breastfeeding Committee and USLCA's representative to the US Department of Agriculture's Breastfeeding Promotion Consortium. She sits on the Board of Directors of the US Lactation Consultant Association (USLCA), the Massachusetts Breastfeeding Coalition, and Baby Friendly USA. She is a frequent speaker and the author of over 100 publications on breastfeeding.

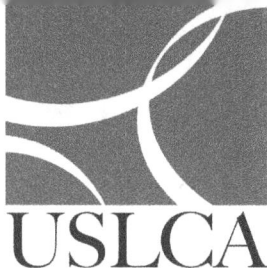

Does Lanolin Use Increase the Risk for Infection in Breastfeeding Women?

Bethany Certa Sasaki, RN, IBCLC, RLC[1]
Katrina Pinkerton, ICCE, IBCLC, RLC[2]
Angelia Leipelt, ICCE, CLEC, IBCLC, RLC[3]

Keywords: Nipple pain, lanolin, bacterial infection, fungal infection

Background: Use of lanolin has become a breast-feeding cultural norm, although the evidence is conflicting on its safety and efficacy. Little to no evidence is available on the relationship between lanolin and infection.

Methods: This is a feasibility study, using case-control, retrospective chart review, examining lanolin use and the development signs and

1   nursebethany@yahoo.com
2   katrina.pinkerton-lloyd@yale.edu
3   leipeltfamily@att.net

symptoms of nipple or breast infection in breast-feeding mothers with nipple pain. Fungal infection versus bacterial infection was suspected according to the corresponding effective treatment.

Results: Lanolin users were suspected to have a 62% infection rate, as compared to non-lanolin users at 18%, odds ratio = 7.5 (95% CI = 2.4–23.4). Although not significant, fungal infection may be more frequent than bacterial infection based on effective corresponding treatment.

Conclusion: A randomized controlled trial is called for to determine if frequent lanolin use increases the risk of nipple or breast infection.

Breastfeeding women may experience nipple and breast infections causing pain severe enough to alter the breast-feeding relationship. Nipple pain and nipple wound healing are areas of nonconsensus among medical and lactation professionals, which may result in delay of symptom relief, endangering the likelihood of continued breastfeeding (Wilson-Clay & Hoover, 2008).

Moist wound healing, usually by applying lanolin after every feeding, is a common recommendation for nipple trauma (Betzold, 2005). However, the association between lanolin and infections has not been established. Does lanolin use by breastfeeding women increase the risk of infection? Does it specifically increase the risk of fungal infection? Could antibiotic use further increase this risk?

Background

Nipple Areolar Complex

The nipple and areola are self-lubricating structures. The nipple is composed of mesenchymal smooth muscle cells covered in epithelial cells and contains sebaceous and apocrine sweat glands (Lawrence & Lawrence, 2011). Like all skin, the nipple and areola breathe and perspire. The areola is circumscribed with Montgomery glands, which secrete lubrication to protect the entire nippleareolar complex (Lawrence & Lawrence, 2011). The nipple and areola do not require creams and lotions because these substances will reduce the amount of air circulation to the skin, and secretions from the Montgomery glands may provide the baby with a smell aiding in nipple location (Lauwers & Swisher, 2010). The lymph system of the breast drains from the cutaneous area through the breast to the parasternal and axillary nodes (Lawrence & Lawrence, 2011).

Box 1. Clinical Presentation

Amy D. is a 26-year-old G1P1 breastfeeding Delilah, a 3-week-old girl. Latch had been uncomfortable, but tolerable. She presents with worsening left nipple pain. The right nipple is pain free. The left nipple is red, flaky, tender between feedings, and cracked, with red streaks extending into the breast tissue. On history, she was treated with antibiotics in labor and uses lanolin after every feeding. The lactation consultant improved latch on the left side, recommended keeping the nipple clean and dry, and referred to the OB for evaluation, where she was prescribed dicloxacillin. The symptoms subsided for 1 week and returned bilaterally with painful, red, cracked nipples.

Infections

There are multiple causes of nipple infections and mastitis. This article will focus on two common pathogens: *Candida albicans* and *Staphylococcus aureus*. Candida colonizes the skin, gastrointestinal tract, and vagina; favoring warm, moist areas; and is found in the mouths of most infants (Osterman & Rahm, 2000). With a 32% average cesarean-section rate nationally (Menacker, 2010), and 10%–30% of women being Group B *Streptococcus* positive (Centers for Disease Control and Prevention, 2010), it could be calculated that approximately 30%–60% of women are receiving intravenous antibiotic therapy at the time of birth, placing them at risk for secondary fungal infections.

The incidence of vulvovaginal candidiasis after exposure to antibiotics is well established (Spinillo, Capuzzo, Acciano, De Santolo, & Zara, 1999) as well as the incidence of candiduria (Weinberger, 2003).

Candida infection makes the epidermis friable; skin breakdown may occur and barrier protection is lost (Wilson-Clay & Hoover, 2008). Fetherston (1998) found that candidiasis led to infectious mastitis in most cases. Dennis, Allen, McCormick, and Renfrew (2008) explain that breakdown in the tissue integrity of the nipple or areola expose the breast to symptoms of fungal or bacterial infection, including symptoms of a *Candida* infection. Osterman and Rahm (2000) found that women experiencing lactation mastitis were most frequently colonized with *S. aureus*. It is noteworthy that *methicillin-resistant S.*

aureus (MRSA) is also known to infect the breast and cause abscesses (Wilson-Clay, 2008).

Lanolin

Lanolin is produced by extracting sebaceous gland secretions from the wool of sheep. Various brands of lanolin nipple cream are sold at retailers and dispensed by healthcare personnel for breastfeeding mothers as a treatment for sore and cracked nipples. The use of lanolin as a nipple treatment has been normalized by retail marketing and healthcare providers. In a breastfeeding handout by the American College of Obstetricians and Gynecologists (ACOG, 2011), women are instructed to *apply 100% pure lanolin to your nipples after feeding* to *keep breasts healthy*.

The Food and Drug Administration (FDA) has not approved lanolin cream specifically for use on nipples, specifies that it is not for oral use and has not tested if it is fully absorbed into skin (Department of Health and Human Services, 2003). Purified lanolin products are marketed to breastfeeding mothers' claim to *soothe and protect mom's sore, cracked nipples,* and state their product is *completely safe for baby* (Lansinoh Laboratories, 2013).

Literature Review

Evidence regarding the effectiveness of lanolin is inconsistent. Studies that examine the relationship between lanolin use and breast infection as the main variable were not found. Studies on lanolin that incidentally measure infection report inconsistent findings. Some report more infections in lanolin groups, others in hydrogel, placebo, or expressed-breast-milk groups.

Dodd and Chalmers (2003) compared hydrogel dressings to lanolin, using 86 patient participants from two hospitals in separate locations within the U.S. They found eight incidences of mastitis and andidiasis, all from the lanolin group, with no infections in the group using hydrogel dressings. Although the eight incidences of infection were considered within normal limits, because nipple damage often leads to infection, the statistical analysis suggested that lanolin use was correlated with breast infection.

Brent, Rudy, Redd, Rudy, and Roth (1998) found the opposite. They compared hydrogel dressings to lanolin plus breast shells, measuring healing and pain. The lanolin-plus-breast-shells group had better results. However, patients with breast infections were excluded from the study, which was ended early because of a high rate of infections in the experimental group.

Melli et al. (2007) conducted a randomized controlled trial treating primiparous breastfeeding women's nipples with peppermint oil gel, lanolin ointment, and placebo gels to prevent nipple damage and also concluded that nipple damage was best prevented using peppermint-oil-gel treatment and was more likely to occur among women using lanolin or placebo gel, although there was no statistical significance between the lanolin and peppermint groups. Infection was seen in the placebo group only.

A study by Abou-Dakn, Fluhr, Gensch, and Wockel (2011) showed that lanolin was more effective than expressed breast milk in reducing nipple pain and promoting tissue healing. Bacterial cultures were taken at enrollment, which grew physiologic skin flora and were not significantly different between the two groups. There were cases of mastitis in the expressed-breast-milk group, but not the lanolin group. However, no statistical analysis is given.

Dennis, Schottle, Hodnett, and McQueen (2012) evaluated the effectiveness of All Purpose Nipple Ointment (APNO) versus lanolin on damaged nipples. They found lanolin to be superior to APNO using a double-blind randomized controlled trial. Both mastitis and nipple *Candida* symptoms were measured at 12 weeks by self-report. Mastitis was reported in 4.1% of the APNO group and 2.7% of the lanolin group. *Candida* symptoms were reported in 8.1% of the APNO group and 11.0% of the lanolin group. This difference was not statistically significant.

Method

Sample

This is a feasibility study, using chart review to examine lanolin use and the development of signs and symptoms of nipple or breast infections in breastfeeding mothers with nipple pain. Fungal infection versus bacterial infection was suspected according to the corresponding effective treatment. A retrospective case-control study was done using 131 charts, spanning a 2-year period, from the private lactation consulting practice of an International Board Certified Lactation Consultant (IBCLC). Confidence intervals were calculated using Epi Info.

Participants whose charts were included in the sample had already signed an optional consent allowing their anonymous clinical information to be used for research. Permission to perform the chart review was granted by the Dignity Health Sacramento-Sierra Regional IRB. All participants were adult, breastfeeding mothers, living within a 50-mile radius of Sacramento, California, between 2010 and 2012.

Data Collection

Four main data points were extracted:

a. nipple pain or trauma,

b. lanolin use,

c. development of signs and symptoms of nipple or breast infection, and

d. resolution of these symptoms with antifungals, antibiotics, or nipple hygiene.

Nipple pain and trauma were noted by self-report or clinician assessment. Lanolin use was noted if used daily or more frequently. Infection was suspected by the presence of the following symptoms: nipple and areolar erythema with severe pain (burning, stabbing, between feedings), and/or severe breast pain with a fever and malaise. Plugged ducts that resolved mechanically were not suspected to be an infection.

Antifungal treatments included Nystatin, Monistat, Diflucan, gentian violet, and probiotics. Clients being treated for suspected fungal infections treated their baby as well. Antibiotics included dicloxacillin, cefazolin, and other prescription antibiotics. Nipple hygiene included hand washing, rinsing the nipples after feeding sessions, discontinuing topical treatments, and air drying the nipples. Nipple hygiene sometimes involved using coconut oil in place of lanolin, only if the client insisted she needed a topical moisturizer to tolerate breastfeeding.

Results

Of the sample of 131 client charts, 4 were excluded from the study because of insufficient follow-up data, 2 were excluded for plugged ducts, and 1 was excluded for an allergic reaction to lanolin, making the final sample size 124.

The participants were socioeconomically homogeneous, but racially diverse. The population was stratified by nipple pain. Thirty-eight mothers with nipple pain did not use lanolin, and 27 did use lanolin. In the non-lanolin group, 18% (n = 7) developed signs of a nipple or breast infection. In the lanolin group, 62% (n = 17) developed signs of a nipple or breast infection. Odds ratio = 7.5 (95% CI = 2.4–23.4; see Table 1).

Table 1. Development of Nipple or Breast Infection Symptoms		
Groups	Infection	No Infection
Lanolin	17	10
Non-lanolin	7	31

All 17 clients in the lanolin group who developed signs and symptoms of infection were advised to discontinue lanolin. Of the 17, 47% (n = 8) resolved with antifungals, 35% (n = 6) resolved with a combination of antifungals and antibiotics, and 17% (n = 3) resolved with nipple hygiene. One-way ANOVA was not significant (see Table 2).

Table 2. Resolution of Nipple or Breast Infection Symptom in the Lanolin Group	
Resolved With	Lanolin Group
Antifungals	8
Combination of antifungals and antibiotics	6
Nipple hygiene	3

Discussion

The IBCLC should provide evidence-based guidance. The evidence at this time is conflicting and not sufficient to determine if lanolin use is related to infection. Although some clinicians believe that wound healing may be hastened with lanolin, the wound itself is an entry point for pathogens. The authors hypothesized that lanolin and moist-wound healing may be providing an environment ideal for bacterial and fungal growth. Research is needed to evaluate this relationship and to examine causation. The potential for infection must be ruled out prior to making lanolin standard practice.

Although our sample was too small to show significance, many of the participants had symptoms of fungal infection. Research is needed to determine if lanolin applied to nipples, coated with a baby's oral flora, becomes a growth medium for *Candida*.

Clinicians treating women for nipple and breast infections should obtain a history of intrapartum antibiotic use. Altered flora from antibiotics, plus a history of frequent lanolin use, should trigger an assessment for nipple or ductal candidiasis.

Conclusion

Our preliminary data suggest that lanolin use may increase the risk for infection. Fungal infection was suspected to be the most frequent pathogen. This study is limited by the small convenience sample. Also, we were unable to control for hand hygiene; because lanolin is applied with the fingers, this is an important confounder.

This data shows the feasibility of a larger randomized controlled trial to determine the relationship between lanolin use and infection. Women would be enrolled prenatally and assigned to a group at birth. One group would be assigned to lanolin use after each feeding, a second group assigned to no topical treatments, and both followed for development of infection. The groups should be stratified by broken skin, peripartum exposure to antibiotics, and type of infection. Standardized instructions, such as hand hygiene and standardized lactation support, should be given to both groups. The results of such a study would greatly benefit the evidence base for lactation consultants.

References

Abou-Dakn, M., Fluhr, J., Gensch, M., & Wockel, A. (2011). Positive effect of HPA lanolin versus expressed breastmilk on painful and damaged nipples during lactation. *Skin Pharmacology Physiology*, 24, 27–35..

American College of Obstetricians and Gynecologists. (2011). *Frequently asked questions: Breastfeeding your baby.* Retrieved from http://www.acog.org/~/media/For%20Patients/faq029.pdf

Betzold, C. (2005). Infections of the mammary ducts in the breastfeeding mother. *The Journal for Nurse Practitioners*, 15–21. http://dx.doi.org/10.1016/j.nurpra.2005.06.001

Brent, N., Rudy, S. J., Redd, B., Rudy, T. E., & Roth, L. A. (1998). Sore nipples in breast-feeding women: A clinical trial of wound dressings vs. conventional care. *Archives of Pediatric and Adolescent Medicine*, 152(11), 1077–1082.

Centers for Disease Control and Prevention. (2010). *Prevention of perinatal group b streptococcal disease.* Retrieved from http://www.cdc.gov/mmwr/pdf/rr/rr5910.pdf

Dennis, C., Allen, K., McCormick, F., & Renfrew, M. (2008). *Interventions for treating painful nipples among breastfeeding women* (Protocol), (4), CD007366. http://dx.doi.org/10.1002/14651858.CD007366. Cochrane Database of Systematic Reviews(4).

Dennis, C., Schottle, N., Hodnett, E., & McQueen, K. (2012). An all purpose nipple ointment versus lanolin in treating damaged nipples in breastfeeding women: A randomized controlled trial. *Breastfeeding Medicine*, 7(6), 473–479. http://dx.doi.org/10.1089/bfm.2011.0121

Department of Health and Human Services. (2003). *Skin protectant drug products for over-the-counter human use* [Final Monograph]. Food and Drug Administration 21 CFR Parts 310, 347, and 352 [Docket Nos. 78N–0021 and 78N–021P] RIN 0910–AA01. Retrieved from http://www.fda.gov/downloads/Drugs/ DevelopmentApprovalProcess/DevelopmentResources/Over-the-CounterOTCDrugs/StatusofOTCRulemakings/ucm091520.pdf

Dodd, V., & Chalmers, C. (2003). Comparing the use of hydrogel dressings to lanolin ointment in lactating mothers. *Journal of Obstetrical Gynecological and Neonatal Nurses, 32*, 486–494.

Fetherston, K. (1998). Risk factors for lactation mastitis. *Journal of Human Lactation, 14*(2), 101–109.

Lansinoh Laboratories. (2013). *HPA lanolin*. Retrieved from https://www.lansinoh.com/products/hpa-lanolin

Lauwers, J., & Swisher, A. (2010). *Counseling the nursing mother* (5th ed.). Sudbury, MA: Jones and Bartlett.

Lawrence, R., & Lawrence, R. (2011). *Breastfeeding: A guide for the medical profession* (7th ed.). Philadelphia, PA: Elsevier Mosby.

Melli, M., Rashidi, M., Nokhoodchi, A., Tagavi, S., Farzadi, L., Sadaghat, K., . . . Sheshvan, M. (2007). A randomized trial of peppermint gel, lanolin ointment and placebo gel to prevent nipple crack in primiparous breastfeeding women. *Medical Science Monitor, 13*(9), 406–411.

Menacker, F. (2010). *Recent trends in caesarian delivery in the United States*. Retrieved from http://www.cdc.gov/nchs/data/databriefs/db35.pdf

Osterman, K., & Rahm, V. (2000). Lactation mastitis: Bacterial ultivation of breast milk, symptoms, treatment and outcomes. *Journal of Human Lactation, 16*(4), 297–302.

Spinillo, A., Capuzzo, E., Acciano, S., De Santolo, A., & Zara, F. (1999). Effect of antibiotic use on the prevalence of symptomatic vulvovaginal candidiasis. *American Journal of Obstetrics and Gynecology, 180*, 14–17.

Weinberger, M. (2003). Correlation between candiduria and departmental antibiotic use. *Journal of Hospital Infection, 53*(3), 183–186.

Wilson-Clay, B. (2008). Case report of methicillin-resistant staphylococcus aureus (MRSA) mastitis with abscess formation in a breastfeeding woman. *Journal of Human Lactation, 24*, 326–329.

Wilson-Clay, B., & Hoover, K. (2008). *The breastfeeding atlas*. Manchaca TX: LactNews Press.

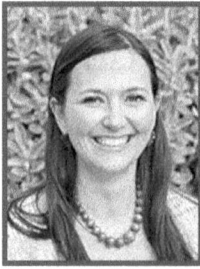

Bethany Certa Sasaki, RN, BSN, IBCLC, RLC, is a registered nurse, an International Board Certified Lactation Consultant, and a graduate student at Frontier Nursing University in the Nurse-Midwifery program. She is kept busy by her two children, her private lactation practice, and filling in as an in-patient lactation consultant at the Mercy Women's Center and as an RN at The Birth Center in Sacramento, CA. This is her first publication.

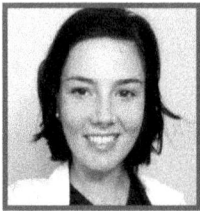

Katrina Pinkerton, ICCE, IBCLC, RLC, has worked as an in-patient lactation consultant for two years and taught childbirth classes for four years in Sacramento Ca. She currently is a student of nurse-midwifery at Yale University, and teaches prenatal and breastfeeding classes to expecting high school students in New Haven, CT.

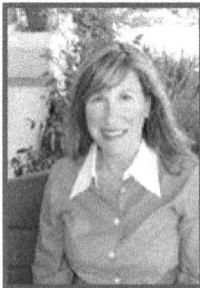

Angelia Leipelt, ICCE, CLEC, IBCLC, RLC, is an International Board Certified Lactation Consultant and International Childbirth Education Association childbirth educator. She works as a lactation consultant for Mercy Women's Center—both in-patient and privately—and teaches breastfeeding and childbirth education in the hospital setting. As the lead lactation consultant for Methodist Hospital in Sacramento, CA, she cares for well newborns, NICU babies, trains medical residents in breastfeeding, and is a member of the Breastfeeding Task Force working toward the Baby-Friendly Hospital Designation.

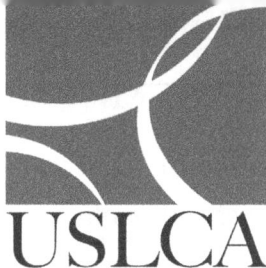

Topical Treatments Used by Breastfeeding Women to Treat Sore and Damaged Nipples

Miranda L. Buck, RN, BA, MPhil, IBCLC, RLC[1]
Lisa H. Amir, MBBS, MMed, PhD, IBCLC, RLC, FABM, FILCA[2]
Susan M. Donath, BSc, MEc, MA[3]

Keywords: Breastfeeding, nipple pain, nipple cream, lanolin

Background: *Nipple pain and trauma are frequent complaints of new mothers, and a variety of treatments have been proposed and investigated for efficacy. Numerous studies have examined the efficacy of nipple creams, but there is no published data describing patterns of use in breastfeeding women.*

1   m.buck@latrobe.edu.au
2   l.amir@latrobe.edu.au
3   susan.donath@mcri.edu.au

Aim: *To describe the use of topical nipple treatments by a cohort of first-time mothers in Australia.*

Methods: *A cohort of 360 nulliparous women were recruited in Melbourne, Australia, and the question, "In the last week, have you used any creams or ointments on your nipples?" was included in a questionnaire on breastfeeding practices administered at 6 time points.*

Results: *In the first week after giving birth, 91% (307/336) of women used a topical treatment on their nipples. The most popular treatment was purified lanolin, with nearly three quarters of women (250/336) reporting its use. At 8 weeks postpartum, 37% (129/345) continued to use topical treatments, and 94% (320/340) of women continued to breastfeed.*

Conclusion: *Widespread use of topical nipple creams is concerning not only because it may indicate a high rate of nipple pain, but also because this is a disruption to the natural environment where the newborn is establishing breastfeeding.*

Nipple pain and damage are common problems for postpartum women. Our recent study in Melbourne, Australia, found 80% of new mothers experience nipple pain in the postpartum period, with rates little changed since the first studies were conducted in the U.S. in the 1950s, despite many changes in the culture and practices of postnatal care (Buck, Amir, Cullinane, & Donath, 2014; Newton, 1952).

We found no difference in pain between women who had vaginal or caesarean birth (Buck et al., 2014). Nipple pain is the second most common reason women give for weaning, and the most common for discontinuing breastfeeding before leaving hospital (Lewallen et al., 2006; Li, Fein, Chen, & Grummer-Strawn, 2008; Scott, Landers, Hughes, & Binns, 2001; Tucker, Wilson, & Samandari, 2011). Qualitative studies of women's breastfeeding experiences have consistently found that nipple pain has been an unexpectedly unpleasant burden on new mothers, and which has in some cases negatively affect a woman's relationship with her baby (Amir, 2004; Kelleher, 2006; Williamson, Leeming, Lyttle, & Johnson, 2012).

The application of various preparations to soothe and heal nipples is widely recommended (Nancey, 2008; Porter & Schach, 2004; Rennie, Cowie, Hindin, & Jewell, 2009; Walker, 2013). Traditional remedies, such as onions, peppermint water, and olive oil, are also used by breast-feeding women (Akcan & Ozkiraz, 2012; Gungor et al., 2012; Sayyah Melli et al., 2007), and a recent survey of lactation instructors in the U.S. found that 65% recommend folk remedies (Schaffir & Czapla, 2012).

There are several commercially prepared nipple creams available in Australia marketed for the treatment and prevention of sore nipples. Some topical nipple treatments have been shown to reduce pain and improve healing, which may help women's experience of breastfeeding and support them in persisting to find solutions to their breastfeeding problems (Lochner, Livingston, & Judkins, 2009).

However, two systematic reviews of interventions for nipple pain and trauma in breastfeeding women, Morland-Schultz and Hill (2005) and Vieira, Bachion, Mota, and Munari (2013), concluded that there is a lack of evidence as to the efficacy of any treatment because the studies which have been undertaken to date have lacked rigor.

This article presents prospective data from breast-feeding women documenting their use of nipple treatments over the first 8 postpartum weeks, using data collected in the *Candida* and *Staphylococcus* Transmission: Longitudinal Evaluation (CASTLE) study. The main aim of the CASTLE study was to determine whether *Staphylococcus aureus* or *Candida albicans* is the primary organism involved in breast thrush in lactating women, and further details are available in the published protocol and results (Amir et al., 2011, 2013).

Methods

Setting

Women were recruited from two hospitals in Melbourne, Australia: The Royal Women's Hospital (RWH), a public tertiary women's hospital in Melbourne, and Frances Perry House (FPH), a private hospital located on the same site. RWH has been accredited as Baby Friendly since 1995, and both hospitals have dedicated lactation support services. There is an onsite public pharmacy, separate from the hospital pharmacy, which sells a variety of commercial nipple ointments.

Study Sample

A prospective cohort of 360 nulliparous women was recruited between November 2009 and June 2011 (Amir et al., 2011).

Eligibility criteria for the study were 18–50 years of age, nulliparity, $36 weeks pregnant at recruitment, singleton pregnancy, breastfeeding intention for at least 8 weeks postpartum, sufficient proficiency in English to complete written questionnaires and a telephone interview, and residing #16 km from Melbourne Central Business District. Criteria for exclusion were medical conditions that do not allow breastfeeding, breast reduction surgery, dermatitis on nipple during pregnancy, under care of the Women's Alcohol and Drug Service, and under care of mental health service or social worker.

Data Collection

The participants completed a questionnaire about their breastfeeding practices in hospital and at Weeks, 1, 2, 3, 4, and 8. The question asked was, *In the last week, have you used any creams or ointments on your nipples?*

There were several options of types of topical treatment and a space to write any other treatments used. Any comments the participants made about why they were using the treatments during the visits were noted by the researchers; participant study numbers are presented alongside the quotes.

Results

Of the 360 women recruited at 36 weeks gestation, 14 were lost from the study, and there was data available for 346; 154 from RWH and 192 from FPH.

The mean age was 32.7 years with a range of 19–44, and the caesarean rate was 45% (156/346). This was a highly educated sample of women, with 77% (267/346) having a tertiary degree or higher. The majority of the women were married or living with their partner (332/346). The mean intention to breastfeed was 9.7 months (range 1–24 months). At 8 weeks, 80% of the babies were fully breastfed, and 94% (320/340) were receiving any breast milk.

In the first week after birth, 91% (307/336) of women were using some form of nipple treatment (see Table 1). By far the most popular choice of treatment was purified lanolin; 74% (250/336) of postpartum women were using lanolin at Week 1, almost half were using it after 4 weeks and at 8 weeks 26% (89/345).

Overall, 18 distinct commercial treatments were found to be in use, and one woman used olive oil. Early in the study period, Weeks 1–4, hydrogel dressings were used by up to 12% (40/336) of women for the treatment of cracked and damaged nipples, but use of hydrogel dressings had been discontinued by 8 weeks.

Table 1. Treatments Used By Week

Type of Treatment	Hospital (n = 338) n (%)	Week 1 (n = 336) n (%)	Week 2 (n = 336) n (%)	Week 3 (n = 326) n (%)	Week 4 (n = 323) n (%)	Week 8 (n = 345) n (%)
Purified lanolin	103 (30)	250 (74)	220 (65)	178 (56)	155 (48)	89 (26)
Antifungal cream	0	1 (0.3)	3 (1)	1 (0.3)	2 (1)	1 (0.3)
Antifungal gel	0	1 (0.3)	8 (2)	12 (4)	17 (5)	26 (8)
Gentian Violet	0	0	0	0	0	2 (1)
Antibiotic ointment	1 (0.3)	0	0	2 (1)	0	1 (0.3)
Combination ointment	1 (0.3)	0	2 (1)	6 (2)	4 (1)	1 (0.3)
Hydrogel dressing	11 (3)	40 (12)	31 (9)	18 (6)	17 (5)	0
Lucas' Pawpaw Ointment[a]	2 (1)	6 (2)	2 (1)	6 (2)	1 (0.3)	6 (2)
Other[b]	4 (1)	9 (3)	6 (2)	11 (3)	9 (3)	3 (1)

[a]Lucas' Pawpaw Ointment is an Australian product containing petroleum jelly and *Carica papaya*.

[b]A number of other creams were used by individual women: Aveda Nipple Care Balm, Bepanthen, Betadine Antiseptic Ointment, Calendula cream, Gentian Violet (two women in week 8), Mustela Nursing Comfort Balm, Nuk Nipple Cream, olive oil, Palmer's Cocoa Butter Nursing Cream, phytoseptic (Golden Seal; *Hydrastis Canadensis*), QV cream, Vaseline, Weleda Nipple Care Cream.

The following comments are examples of the notes taken by researchers during their visits with the participants to collect data:

Between wk 4 & 5 postpartum participant had stabbing breast pain. Infant had white coating on tongue. Participant's sister-in-law (midwife) suggested she may have nipple thrush. Participant went to pharmacist who also suggested nipple thrush and gave participant Daktarin gel [miconazole]. Participant used Daktarin gel for 3 days on her nipple every feed. The breast pain went away after this time. White coating also disappeared from baby's tongue. (Participant FPH190) 3 wk ago participant thought she had nipple thrush. She thought her baby had oral thrush. She brought her baby to GP who did not diagnose oral thrush, but prescribed Daktarin gel for mother's nipples and baby's mouth as a precaution. Participant used Daktarin on her nipples for a week and intermittently since then. (Participant RWH82) Participant had stabbing breast pain in right breast this week. Given Daktarin oral gel. GP told her to use it on the right nipple only. Not putting it in the baby's mouth. (Participant FPH104) GP prescribed antibiotics and Daktarin gel for suspected mastitis. (Participant RWH110)

Antifungal gel usage was observed as an increasing trend over the duration of the study, from one woman in Week 1 to 26 (8%) in week 8. This rising prevalence was not seen for combination, antibiotic, or non-medicated creams.

In keeping with this rise in antifungal use over the study period, two women had begun to use Gentian Violet by the end of the study. Over the entire study, antifungal gels were used by 47 (14%) individual women. Two women used antifungal gel from Weeks 2 to 8, and four women (1%) from Weeks 3 to 8.

Discussion

The strengths of this study are that it was a prospective study with high retention, and the women reported all usage of topical nipple treatments in the first 8 weeks of breastfeeding.

There was a sharp increase in use of treatments between data collected in hospital and at the end of Week 1. It is possible that when they were presented with the list of creams that may have been used in the first few days after birth, it suggested to the women that they should or could be using a cream, and therefore artificially inflated the prevalence.

This study is not able to evaluate how successful the strategies were or why the women chose those particular products, and we did not ask if they were advised to use them by a healthcare professional. We did not specifically ask the women if they had been applying breast milk to their nipples or about their hygiene practices generally.

Many of the participants were recruited in the breast-feeding education classes provided by the hospital, and lanolin is was likely to have been recommended in those classes and also by the midwives on the antenatal wards (A. Moorhead, Clinical Midwife Consultant, personal communication, June 16, 2014).

Intervention Strategies for Mothers With Sore Nipples

Most women experience some initial difficulties with pain and damage during the early days of breastfeeding. When pain and damage interfere with the establishment of breastfeeding, specific and holistic treatment is warranted. Brodribb (2012) recommends the following principles of general management:

- Offer the least sore nipple first.

- Induce letdown before bringing the baby to the breast.

- Suggest baby-led latch or an upright koala hold.

- Encourage small frequent feeds to prevent engorgement.

- Apply warm compresses immediately post feeds for 5 minutes.

- A moist wound healing environment between feeds will reduce pain and speed wound healing.

Nipple Care During the Early Postpartum Period

Recommendations for nipple care vary enormously and can be conflicting; women are variously advised to wash their nipples with soap, or with nothing but plain water, to apply breast milk, to apply creams, of the benefits of a moist healing environment, or to air dry their nipples and frequently change breast pads to prevent dampness

(Australian Breastfeeding Association, 2011; Newman & Kernerman, 2009; Walker, 2013). This is the first study to prospectively explore the use of topical therapies by breast-feeding women. Over the 8 weeks of the study, a pattern of almost universal use of some form of treatment was seen in the early weeks decreasing over time.

Wound Healing and Lanolin Use

Wound healing can be described in terms of three stages—*inflammation, granulation,* and *remodeling*—and is influenced by many factors including age, sex hormones, medications, stress, and nutrition (Guo & DiPietro, 2010; Kondo & Ishida, 2010). The lactating woman's nipple is a particularly challenging area to support in terms of healing because of the necessity to keep using the tissue and concerns for the infant's safety when topical medications may be ingested.

Nearly three quarters of this cohort applied purified lanolin to their nipples in the first week of breastfeeding. Lanolin is extracted from sheep wool and is chemically a wax "ultrarefined" to remove free lanolin alcohols to a level lower than 1.5% (Abou-Dakn, Fluhr, Gensch, & Wöckel, 2011). It has been successfully used for several therapeutic purposes including healing anal fissures in children and preventing lip breakdown in adults undergoing chemotherapy (Büyükyavuz, Savas, & Duman, 2010; Santos et al., 2013). Chvapil, Gaines, and Gilman (1988), in their detailed study of lanolin and wound healing in piglets, suggested that lanolin may promote an inflammatory response, which encourages re-epithelialization. On a cellular level, the promotion of healing is better than a plain gauze dressing.

Purified lanolin provides a moist healing environment and has been compared to other treatments for sore nipples, and shown to be helpful in reducing pain and supporting healing, but most studies have been small (Coca & Abrao, 2008; Gungor et al., 2012; Vieira et al., 2013). Although concerns have been voiced that lanolin may be associated with an increased risk of infection (Sasaki, Pinkerton, & Leipelt, 2014), Dennis, Schottle, Hodnett, and McQueen (2012) found that in their Toronto study of 151 women, those using lanolin had higher breastfeeding rates at 12 weeks postpartum, and had a significantly more pleasant experience of breastfeeding than those using an all-purpose combined cream.

Increased Use of Antifungals During the First 8 Weeks

Over the course of the first 8 weeks postpartum, women's use of lanolin slowly fell, but antifungal treatments were increasingly popular, with 8% (29/346) using some form of antifungal in Week 8, including two women who were prescribed Gentian Violet. Gentian Violet is recommended on the RWH protocol for the treatment of nipple thrush, as a 0.5% aqueous paint, to be applied after breastfeeding twice a day for up to 7 days, when miconazole, nystatin, and fluconazole treatments have failed (RWH, 2013). Comments made by the women on why they were using antifungal gel suggests that some of the use may be preventive and used in tandem with antibiotics for mastitis. Four women (1%) reported using antifungal gel for 4 weeks and two women for six weeks. This prolonged use of antifungal gel is concerning.

Other Topical Treatments

Lucas' Pawpaw ointment is an Australian product containing petroleum jelly and *Carica Papaya* extract, and was used by small numbers of women at each time point. Several of the creams used, Palmer's, QV, and Bepanthen are petroleum-based, and some contain polyethylene glycol ethers, which are not recommended for use on broken skin and known to be irritants (Andersen, 1999).

Phytoseptic ointment, Weleda, and calendula creams were also used by women in this study. There has been an increasing interest in the use of plant-based extracts in wound healing, and several studies have been published that are promising and suggest that many traditional herbal remedies may be useful. Süntar et al. (2011), for example, found that a preparation of sage and oregano oils "displays remarkable wound healing activity" and is both bactericidal and fungicidal. Cinnamon, lemongrass, and peppermint have also suggested as potential novel therapies (Liakos et al., 2014; Sayyah Melli et al., 2007). Coconut oil has been shown to be antifungal, antibacterial, used safely in topical massage of premature babies, and as a useful treatment in the wound healing of burns (Das, Rahman, Chowdhury, Hoq, & Deb, 2013; Nangia, Paul, Chawla, & Deorari, 2008; Ogbolu, Oni, Daini, & Oloko,

2007; Srivastava & Durgaprasad, 2008; Valizadeh, Hosseini, Jafarabadi, & Ajoodanian, 2012).

Hydrogel Dressings

Hydrogel dressings were used by 12% of the women, but use had been discontinued by Week 8 of the study. These dressings are expensive; there has been some concerns raised that although they may reduce pain, they may increase the risk of infection (Benbow & Vardy-White, 2004; Brent, Rudy, Redd, Rudy, & Roth, 1998), and they are not recommended by Vieira et al. (2013) in their systematic review.

Concerns About the Use of Topical Treatments

The mother's breast is the native environment of the newborn baby, and skin-to-skin contact between neonate and mother at birth initiates a cascade of primitive behaviors and reflexes that supports the establishment of both breastfeeding and the mother–infant bond (Barry & Tighe, 2013; Bigelow, Littlejohn, Bergman, & McDonald, 2010; Bramson et al., 2010; Colson, Meek, & Hawdon, 2008; Mahmood, Jamal, & Khan, 2011; Widström et al., 2011).

How well the newborn baby initially seeks out and attaches to the nipple may influence the course of breastfeeding, and this in turn is influenced by the sensory environment at the breast. The smell and feel of their mother's skin varies by birthing and hygiene practices and also according to secretions of Montgomery glands on the nipple (Doucet, Soussignan, Sagot, & Schaal, 2009, 2012;

Preer, Pisegna, Cook, Henri, & Philipp, 2013). It is of some concern that such widespread use of topical creams was found not only because it may indicate a high frequency of nipple pain but also because this is a disruption to the natural environment and experience of breastfeeding for the baby, the consequences of which are unknown.

Conclusion

Nipple pain is a key risk to the continuation breastfeeding and also causes considerable distress to new mothers. The use of topical treatments, notably purified lanolin, for the prevention and treatment of nipple problems in breastfeeding is very common, but what this means for the experience of infants at the breast and the establishment of successful breastfeeding is unknown.

Further research is required to establish both an effective intervention for the prevention of nipple trauma and timely treatment of damaged and sore nipples, which need careful evaluation.

References

Abou-Dakn, M., Fluhr, J. W., Gensch, M., & Wöckel, A. (2011). Positive effect of HPA lanolin versus expressed breastmilk on painful and damaged nipples during lactation. *Skin Pharmacology and Physiology, 24*(1), 27–35.

Akcan, A. B., & Ozkiraz, S. (2012). An unusual traditional practice for damaged nipples during lactation. *Breastfeeding Medicine, 7,* 319.

Amir, L. H. (2004). Test your knowledge. Nipple pain in breastfeeding. *Australian Family Physician, 33*(1–2), 44–45.

Amir, L. H., Cullinane, M., Garland, S. M., Tabrizi, S. N., Donath, S. M., Bennett, C. M., . . . Payne, M. S. (2011). The role of micro–organisms

(Staphylococcus aureus and Candida albicans) in the pathogenesis of breast pain and infection in lactating women: Study protocol. *BMC Pregnancy and Childbirth, 11,* 54.

Amir, L. H., Donath, S. M., Garland, S. M., Tabrizi, S. N., Bennett, C. M., Cullinane, M., & Payne, M. S. (2013). Does Candida and/or Staphylococcus play a role in nipple and breast pain in lactation? A cohort study in Melbourne, Australia. *BMJ Open, 3*(3), e002351.

Andersen, F. A. (1999). Final report on the safety assessment of Ceteth 21,22,23,24,25,26,210,212,214,215,216,220,224,225, 230, and 245. *International Journal of Toxicology, 18*(2 Suppl.), 1–8.

Australian Breastfeeding Association. (2011). *Sore/cracked nipples.* Retrieved from https://www.breastfeeding.asn.au/bf-info/ common-concerns%E2%80%93mum/sore-cracked-nipples

Barry, M., & Tighe, S. M. (2013). Facilitating effective initiation of breastfeeding—A review of the recent evidence base. *British Journal of Midwifery, 21*(5), 312–315.

Benbow, M., & Vardy-White, C. (2004). Study into the effectiveness of MOTHERMATES. *British Journal of Midwifery, 12*(4), 244–248.

Bigelow, A. E., Littlejohn, M., Bergman, N., & McDonald, C. (2010). The relation between early mother–infant skin-to-skin contact and later maternal sensitivity in South African mothers of low birth weight infants. *Infant Mental Health Journal, 31*(3), 358–377.

Bramson, L., Lee, J. W., Moore, E., Montgomery, S., Neish, C., Bahjri, K., & Melcher, C. L. (2010). Effect of early skin-to-skin mother–infant contact during the first 3 hours following birth on exclusive breastfeeding during the maternity hospital stay. *Journal of Human Lactation, 26*(2), 130–137.

Brent, N., Rudy, S. J., Redd, B., Rudy, T. E., & Roth, L. A. (1998). Sore nipples in breastfeeding women: A clinical trial of wound dressings vs conventional care. *Archives of Pediatric and AdolescentMedicine, 152*(11), 1077–1082.

Brodribb, W. (2012). *Breastfeeding management in Australia*: Victoria, Australia: Australian Breastfeeding Association.

Buck, M. L., Amir, L. H., Cullinane, M., & Donath, S. M. (2014). Nipple pain, damage and vasospasm in the first 8 weeks postpartum. *Breastfeeding Medicine, 9*(2), 56–62.

Büyükyavuz, B. I., Savas, Ç., & Duman, L. (2010). Efficacy of lanolin and bovine type I collagen in the treatment of childhood anal fissures: A prospective, randomized, controlled clinical trial. *Surgery Today, 40*(8), 752–756.

Chvapil, M., Gaines, J. A., & Gilman, T. (1988). Lanolin and epidermal growth factor in healing of partial-thickness pig wounds. *Journal of Burn Care & Research, 9*(3), 279–284.

Coca, K. P., & Abrao, A. C. F. V. (2008). An evaluation of the effect of lanolin in healing nipple injuries. *Acta Paulista de Enfermagem, 21*(1), 11–16.

Colson, S. D., Meek, J. H., & Hawdon, J. M. (2008). Optimal positions for the release of primitive neonatal reflexes stimulating breastfeeding. *Early Human Development, 84*(7), 441–449.

Das, S. R., Rahman, A. M., Chowdhury, A. A., Hoq, M. M., & Deb, S. R. (2013). Effect of application of sunflower and coconut oils over the skin of low birth weight babies in prevention of nosocomial infection. *Journal of Dhaka Medical College, 21*(2), 160–165.

Dennis, C.-L., Schottle, N., Hodnett, E., & McQueen, K. (2012). An all-purpose nipple ointment versus lanolin in treating painful damaged nipples in breastfeeding women: A randomized controlled trial. *Breastfeeding Medicine, 7*(6), 473–479.

Doucet, S., Soussignan, R., Sagot, P., & Schaal, B. (2009). The secretion of areolar (Montgomery's) glands from lactating women elicits selective, unconditional responses in neonates. *PLoS One, 4*(10), e7579.

Doucet, S., Soussignan, R., Sagot, P., & Schaal, B. (2012). An overlooked aspect of the human breast: Areolar glands in relation with breastfeeding pattern, neonatal weight gain, and the dynamics of lactation. *Early Human Development, 88*(2), 119–128.

Gungor, A., Oguz, S., Vurur, G., Gencer, M., Uysal, A., Hacivelioglu, S., . . . Cosar, E. (2012). Comparison of olive oil and lanolin in the prevention of sore nipples in nursing mothers [Letter to the editor]. *Breastfeeding Medicine, 8*(3), 334–335.

Guo, S., & DiPietro, L. A. (2010). Factors affecting wound healing. *Journal of Dental Research, 89*(3), 219–229.

Kelleher, C. M. (2006). The physical challenges of early breastfeeding. *Social Science & Medicine, 63*(10), 2727–2738.

Kondo, T., & Ishida, Y. (2010). Molecular pathology of wound healing. *Forensic Science International, 203*(1–3), 93–98.

Lewallen, L. P., Dick, M. J., Flowers, J., Powell, W., Zickefoose, K. T., Wall, Y. G., & Price, Z. M. (2006). Breastfeeding support and early cessation. *Journal of Obstetric, Gynecologic, and Neonatal Nursing, 35*(2), 166–172.

Li, R., Fein, S. B., Chen, J., & Grummer-Strawn, L. M. (2008). Why mothers stop breastfeeding: Mothers' self-reported reasons for stopping during the first year. *Pediatrics, 122*(Supp. 2), S69–S76.

Liakos, I., Rizzello, L., Scurr, D. J., Pompa, P. P., Bayer, I. S., & Athanassiou, A. (2014). All-natural composite wound dressing films of essential oils encapsulated in sodium alginate with antimicrobial properties. *International Journal of Pharmaceutics*, 463(2), 137–145.

Lochner, J. E., Livingston, C. J., & Judkins, D. Z. (2009). Clinical inquiries: Which interventions are best for alleviating nipple pain in nursing mothers? *Journal of Family Practice*, 58(11), 612a–612c.

Mahmood, I., Jamal, M., & Khan, N. (2011). Effect of mother-infant early skin-to-skin contact on breastfeeding status: A randomized controlled trial. *Journal of the College of Physicians and Surgeons Pakistan*, 21(10), 601–605.

Morland-Schultz, K., & Hill, P. D. (2005). Prevention of and therapies for nipple pain: A systematic review. *Journal of Obstetric, Gynecologic & Neonatal Nursing*, 34(4), 428–437.

Nancey, J. S. (2008). Breastfeeding 'struggles': Care and management for sore and cracked nipples. *MIDIRS Midwifery Digest*, 18(4), 561–564.

Nangia, S., Paul, V., Chawla, D., & Deorari, A. (2008). Topical coconut oil application reduces transepidermal water loss in preterm very low birth weight neonates: A randomized clinical trial. *Pediatrics*, 121(Suppl. 2), S139.

Newman, J., & Kernerman, E. (2009). *Sore nipples*. Retrieved from http://www.nbci.ca/index.php?option=com_content&id=48:sore-nipples&Itemid=17

Newton, N. (1952). Nipple pain and nipple damage: Problems in the management of breast feeding. *Journal of Pediatrics*, 41(4), 411–423.

Ogbolu, D., Oni, A., Daini, O., & Oloko, A. (2007). In vitro antimicrobial properties of coconut oil on *Candida* species inIbadan, Nigeria. *Journal of Medicinal Food*, 10(2), 384–387.

Porter, J., & Schach, B. (2004). Treating sore, possibly infected nipples. *Journal of Human Lactation*, 20(2), 221–222.

Preer, G., Pisegna, J. M., Cook, J. T., Henri, A.-M., & Philipp, B. L. (2013). Delaying the bath and in-hospital breastfeeding rates. *Breastfeeding Medicine*, 8, 485–490.

Rennie, A. M., Cowie, J., Hindin, P. K., & Jewell, S. (2009). The management of nipple pain and/or trauma associated with breastfeeding. *Best Practice*, 13(4), 17–20.

Santos, P. S., Tinoco-Araujo, J. E., Souza, L. M., Ferreira, R., Ikoma, M. R., Razera, A. P., & Santos, M. M. (2013). Efficacy of HPA

Lanolin® in treatment of lip alterations related to chemotherapy. *Journal of Applied Oral Science, 21*(2), 163–166.

Sasaki, B. C., Pinkerton, K., & Leipelt, A. (2014). Does lanolin use increase the risk for infection in breastfeeding women? *Clinical Lactation, 5*(1), 28–32.

Sayyah Melli, M., Rashidi, M. R., Delazar, A., Madarek, E., Kargar Maher, M. H., Ghasemzadeh, A., . . . Tahmasebi, Z. (2007). Effect of peppermint water on prevention of nipple cracks in lactating primiparous women: A randomized controlled trial. *International Breastfeeding Journal, 2*, 7.

Schaffir, J., & Czapla, C. (2012). Survey of lactation instructors on folk traditions in breastfeeding. *Breastfeeding Medicine, 7*(4), 230–233.

Scott, J. A., Landers, M. C. G., Hughes, R. M., & Binns, C. W. (2001). Psychosocial factors associated with the abandonment of breastfeeding prior to hospital discharge. *Journal of Human Lactation, 17*(1), 24–30.

Srivastava, P., & Durgaprasad, S. (2008). Burn wound healing property of *Cocos nucifera*: An appraisal. *Indian Journal of Pharmacology, 40*(4), 144–146.

Süntar, I., Akkol, E. K., Keles, H., Oktem, A., Baser, K. H. C., & Yesilada, E. (2011). A novel wound healing ointment: A formulation of *Hypericum perforatum* oil and sage and oregano essential oils based on traditional Turkish knowledge. *Journal of Ethnopharmacology, 134*(1), 89–96.

The Royal Women's Hospital. (2013). *Breast & nipple thrush*. Retrieved from https://www.thewomens.org.au/health-information/breastfeeding/breastfeeding-problems/breast-and-nipple-thrush/

Tucker, C. M., Wilson, E. K., & Samandari, G. (2011). Infant feeding experiences among teen mothers in North Carolina: Findings from a mixed-methods study. *International Breastfeeding Journal, 6*, 14.

Valizadeh, S., Hosseini, M. B., Jafarabadi, M. A., & Ajoodanian, N. (2012). The effects of massage with coconut and sunflower oils on oxygen saturation of premature infants with respiratory distress syndrome treated with nasal continuous positive airway pressure. *Journal of Caring Sciences, 1*(4), 191–199.

Vieira, F., Bachion, M. M., Mota, D. D., & Munari, D. B. (2013). A systematic review of the interventions for nipple trauma in breastfeeding mothers. *Journal of Nursing Scholarship, 45*(2), 116–125.

Walker, M. (2013). Are there any cures for sore nipples? *Clinical Lactation, 4*(3), 106–115.

Widström, A. M., Lilja, G., Aaltomaa-Michalias, P., Dahllöf, A., Lintula, M., & Nissen, E. (2011). Newborn behaviour to locate the breast when skin-to-skin: A possible method for enabling early self-regulation. *Acta Paediatrica, 100*(1), 79–85.

Williamson, I., Leeming, D., Lyttle, S., & Johnson, S. (2012). 'It should be the most natural thing in the world': Exploring firsttime mothers' breastfeeding difficulties in the UK using audiodiaries and interviews. *Maternal & Child Nutrition, 8*(4), 434–447.

Ethics: This study was approved by the La Trobe University Human Ethics Committee (06–078), Human Research Ethics Committee of The Royal Women's Hospital (06/41); Human Research Ethics Committee of the University of Melbourne (1033949), and Medical Advisory Committee at Frances Perry House.

Funding: This study received financial support from the National Health and Medical Research Council (project grant 541907, equipment grant, Health Professional Training Fellowship [LHA]), Helen Macpherson Smith Trust, Faculty Research Grant, Faculty of Health Sciences, La Trobe University. MLB has a Faculty of Health Sciences, La Trobe University, Dean's Scholarship.

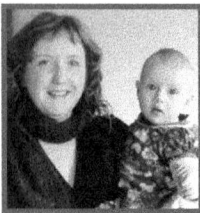

Miranda L. Buck, RN, BA, MPhil, IBCLC, RLC, is a neonatal nurse and International Board Certified Lactation Consultant. She works as a lactation consultant at The Royal Women's Hospital in Melbourne, and is a PhD candidate at the Judith Lumley Centre, La Trobe University. A recipient of the dean's scholarship in 2010, Ms. Buck is investigating women's experiences of breastfeeding problems and nipple pain using data collected in the CASTLE project.

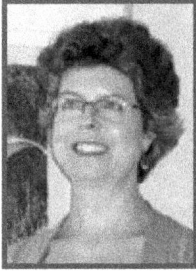

Lisa H. Amir, MBBS, MMed, PhD, IBCLC, RLC, FABM, FILCA, is a general practitioner and lactation consultant. She works in breastfeeding medicine at The Royal Women's Hospital and in private practice. She is a principal research fellow at the Judith Lumley Centre, La Trobe University, Australia. She is the author of over 60 peer-reviewed articles and the editor-in-chief of *International Breastfeeding Journal.*

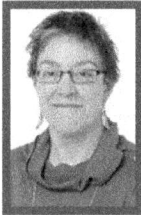

Susan M. Donath, BSc, MEc, MA, is a senior biostatistician and epidemiologist with extensive experience in the design and analysis of quantitative health-related research, perinatal epidemiology, and clinical trials. Susan is an author of more than 130 publications in refereed journals, 70 of which have been published in the last 5 years. These publications cover a wide spectrum of research areas, including laboratory-based, clinical, public health, nursing, and allied health research projects, predominantly in pediatric and women's health.

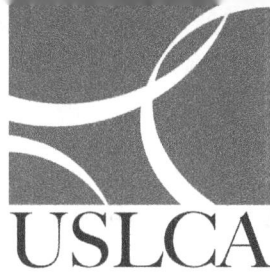

Treating Tongue-Tie
Assessing the Relationship Between Frenotomy and Breastfeeding Symptoms

James W. Ochi, MD[1]

Keywords: Ankyloglossia, breastfeeding, newborns, tongue-tie, frenotomy

Objective: *Ankyloglossia (or "tongue-tie") may increase the risk for newborn breastfeeding symptoms. Lingual frenotomy is the standard treatment for ankyloglossia, but its efficacy at improving the quality of infant breastfeeding has received little formal study. We developed an original 10-question survey of mother and newborn breastfeeding symptoms that are typically observed with ankyloglossia. Possible survey scores ranged from 10 (minimal breastfeeding*

1   jochi@integrativeENT.com Children's ENT of San Diego, Inc., 477 North El Camino Real, Suite C303, Encinitas, CA 92024

symptoms) to a maximum of 50 (extreme symptoms). We predicted that survey scores should decrease after lingual frenotomy.

Method: The survey was administered to mothers of 20 newborns with ankyloglossia, before lingual frenotomy, and about 2 weeks after. The control group consisted of 15 breastfeeding dyads recruited from a breastfeeding support group who filled out the survey twice at 2-week intervals. A 2X2 mixed-methods ANOVA was conducted to test for an interaction between group and time.

Results: Post-hoc analysis of simple effects provided evidence that (a) the frenotomy group had higher survey scores than the control group before intervention and (b) the frenotomy-group survey scores decreased after the intervention. No significant score differences were observed between the frenotomy and control groups after the intervention, and the control group scores did not show a statistically significant decrease over time.

Conclusions: The study provides preliminary evidence for the effectiveness of lingual frenotomy for reducing breastfeeding symptoms associated with ankyloglossia. Furthermore, the study suggests that the use of surveys, such as the one in this study, may help with assessment for ankyloglossia.

Ankyloglossia is increasingly recognized as a cause of breastfeeding problems in newborns.

This entity has been divided into four types based on anatomic location in the oral cavity (Coryllos, Watson Genna, & Salloum, 2004): ankyloglossia Types I and II (Figure 1) are anterior, and Types III and IV are posterior (Table 1).

Lingual frenotomy is typically done for both anterior and posterior conditions (Buryk, Bloom, & Shope, 2011; Hogan, Westcott, & Griffiths, 2005; Hong et al, 2010; O'Callahan, Macary, & Clemente, 2013) and is a straightforward office procedure.

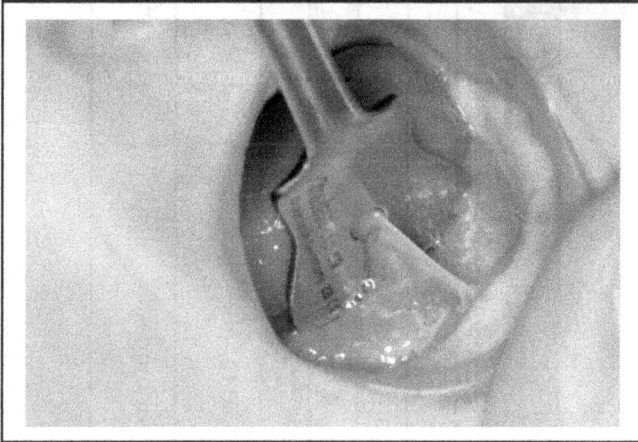

Figure 1. An Example of Ankyloglossia Type II

The lingual frenulum extends inferiorly to just behind the alveolar ridge in this newborn.

Often, babies are able to breastfeed more efficiently, and with less pain to the mother (Dollberg, Botzer, Grunis, & Mimouni, 2006), immediately after the procedure.

Table 1. Anterior and Posterior Ankyloglossia

Ankyloglossia Type	Superior Attachment	Inferior Attachment	Frenulum Characteristics
Anterior			
I	Tongue tip	Alveolar ridge	Often thin, may be elastic
II	2–4 mm behind tip	On or just behind alveolar ridge	Often thin, may be elastic
Posterior			
III	Mid-tongue	Middle of floor of mouth	Usually thicker, more fibrous, and inelastic
IV	Submucosal	Floor of mouth at base of tongue	Usually thick, fibrous, shiny, and inelastic

Although frenotomy is considered the conventional treatment for tongue-tie, its effectiveness at improving the quality of breastfeeding has not been well studied (Amir, James, & Beatty, 2005; Miranda & Milroy, 2010). Therefore, healthcare professional advice and opinions conflict: even in infants with identified ankyloglossia, breastfeeding difficulties were underrecognized and not attributed to tongue-tie (Edmunds, Fulbrook, & Miles, 2013; Edmunds, Miles, & Fulbrook, 2011).

This study thus had two interrelated goals. First and foremost, we wanted to see if infants diagnosed with ankyloglossia experienced improved breastfeeding—as reported by the mother—following lingual frenotomy. Second, we explored—in a preliminary manner—whether or not infants diagnosed with ankyloglossia experienced more breastfeeding symptoms than nondiagnosed infants whose mothers enrolled in a breastfeeding support group.

There are many possible reasons a mother may seek help for breastfeeding. How do mother–infant pairs dealing with ankyloglossia compare to those who simply attend a breastfeeding support group?

Method

Assessment

Breastfeeding symptoms were assessed via the Breastfeeding Symptom Survey (Figure 2) prepared by the author. The survey consists of 10 questions.

Figure 2. Breastfeeding Symptom Survey

Strongly Disagree   Strongly Agree

1. Nursing my baby is painful.	1	2	3	4	5
2. Nursing my baby is frustrating.	1	2	3	4	5
3. My nipples have cracked or bled after nursing.	1	2	3	4	5
4. My nipples are pinched after nursing.	1	2	3	4	5
5. I have cried because of my nursing problems.	1	2	3	4	5
6. My milk supply has gone down.	1	2	3	4	5
7. My baby feeds for long periods of time.	1	2	3	4	5
8. My baby falls asleep at the breast.	1	2	3	4	5
9. My baby has lots of gas.	1	2	3	4	5
10. My baby makes clicking sounds while nursing.	1	2	3	4	5

Total Points = _____

Name of Parent: _____ Name of Baby: _____

Date: __ / __ / __

Total points range from 10 to 50

Each question asks the mother to score, from 1 to 5, whether she or her baby have a particular symptom associated with breastfeeding. The range of possible scores is 10 (suggesting little to no breastfeeding difficulty) to 50 (suggesting extreme breastfeeding difficulties).

The first six questions inquire about symptoms on the part of the mother and the remaining four relate to the newborn. Babies with ankyloglossia may latch ineffectively and often damage the mother's nipples, causing her pain. Milk transfer is impaired, which is frustrating to both mother and baby. Poor milk transfer can lead to engorgement, mastitis, and decreased milk supply (Hazelbaker, 2010).

When milk transfer is reduced, babies need to feed for longer periods (Griffiths, 2004). Fatigue causes the newborn to fall asleep before completing the feeding. Latching problems make the baby prone to swallowing air. Poor latch causes difficulty maintaining an adequate seal and there may be clicking sounds while the baby breastfeeds. Although these symptoms are not exclusive to ankyloglossia, these are the most common concerns expressed by mothers whose babies have ankyloglossia in the author's clinical practice.

Participants and Procedure

Mothers in the intervention group were a convenience sample of patients diagnosed with ankyloglossia from the author's practice.

These were typically patients referred by lactation consultants or pediatricians. Upon arrival, mothers were asked to complete the Breastfeeding Symptom Survey. The author then performed a conventional physical assessment for ankyloglossia using the Coryllos categorization system, which is the method used by the referring lactation community. If an infant was diagnosed with ankyloglossia, the author offered lingual frenotomy as a possible intervention. All participating infants received the lingual frenectomies in the office during the same visit and were allowed to breastfeed immediately after the procedure. A follow-up copy of the Breastfeeding Symptom Survey was mailed to the mothers about 2 weeks later for completion and return.

Volunteer controls were recruited in person from a nearby breastfeeding-support group sponsored by a local hospital. This is an informal discussion group facilitated by a lactation consultant to help mothers who might have questions or concerns about breastfeeding. Mothers at the meetings completed the same survey at recruitment and received a follow-up survey through the mail about 2 weeks later for completion and return.

Results

The Institutional Review Board of Rady Children's Hospital granted approval for this study. There were 20 consecutive mother–infant pairs over 10 weeks from March to June 2012 found whose babies had lingual frenotomy and had completed both the initial and follow-up surveys.

There were 13 infants with Type III ankyloglossia, 3 with Type II, and 2 each with Types I and IV. Four infants had received an unsuccessful lingual frenotomy elsewhere, with no noticeable change in their breastfeeding symptoms before presentation to the author's practice. None of the study patients required revision procedures, and there were no complications from frenectomies performed as part of this study.

There were 24 control subjects invited to participate in the study; 15 of these completed both the initial and follow-up surveys and were included in the control group, and the remaining 9 were excluded.

The following analyses addressed three primary questions. First, we explored the possibility that an age difference between the frenotomy and breastfeeding-support samples might be influencing survey scores. Second, we tested for a change in survey scores in both groups and explored whether or not the two groups varied in their baseline breastfeeding-symptom scores.

Age as a Possible Confounding Variable

Prior to testing the effects of condition (frenotomy intervention vs. breastfeeding support group) and time (Time 1 and Time 2) on the survey scores, we explored the age differences between the control and frenotomy groups. The control group had a mean age of 47.1 days (SD 5 38.0) with a median age of 38 days. The frenotomy group had a mean age of 25.9 days (SD 5 22.1) with a median age of 15 days. Group-age data are summarized using boxplots in Figure 3 to allow the reader to visualize the age composition of the groups.

Distributions were sufficiently normal to compare the group means using an independent samples t-test, $t(20.99)$ = 1.93, p = .07.

Comparison of group age did not reach statistical significance, but there was a trend to older age in the control group. The combination of this trend, visual analysis of the data, and lack of age matching in the study design suggested that age should be considered a possible confounding variable. Although statistical analysis could not remove this design limitation, two additional analyses were conducted to explore age as a possible confounder.

First, we conducted a formal statistical analysis of the correlation between age and survey score. Specifically, infant's initial age on entering the study was correlated with the amount of change observed between the before and after survey scores, $r(33)$ = .07, p = .67, R^2 = .01.

Second, relevant subsets of the control group were visualized to informally assess a possible link between age and change in survey scores. We explored the possibility that the infants in the frenotomy group—being slightly younger on average—may have received high survey scores prior to the treatment because they were younger, and thus their mothers were less experienced with breastfeeding. In this case, we would expect the youngest infants to show the largest decline. The five breastfeeding support group children with the largest decline in survey scores were selected with

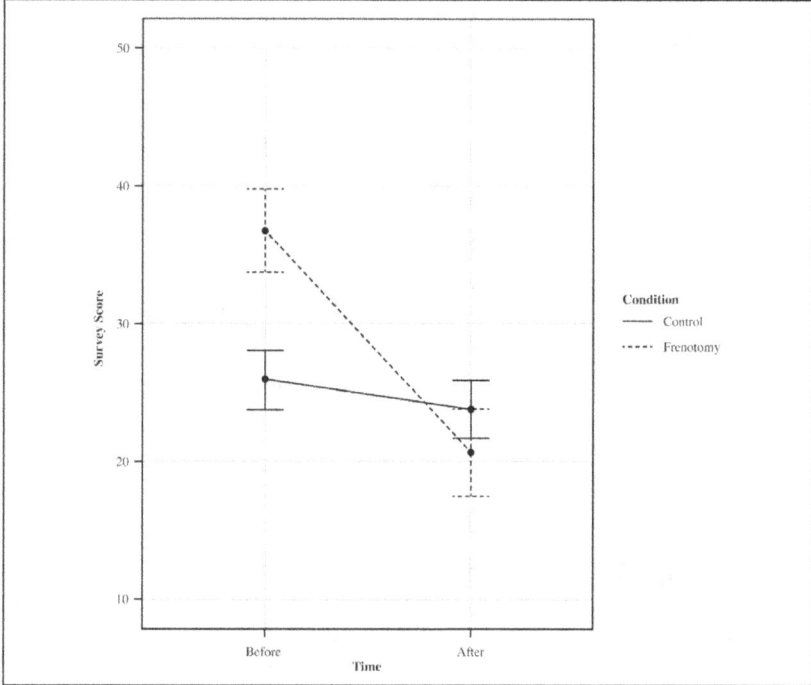

Figure 5. Line Plot of Group Mean Survey Scores

This takes the mean trends shown in Figure 4 and superimposes them over each other to aid in visualizing possible condition by time interactions. The whiskers represent the 95% confidence interval for each mean.

changes in survey scores of -16, -10, -5, -5, and -4. The ages of these children in days at the first survey were 34, 50, 79, 17, and 19, respectively. Only the latter two values fall into an age range comparable to the frenotomy group. In other words, the infants who had the largest decline in survey scores were relatively older. This is the opposite of what we would expect to see if age were a key factor in explaining improvements in infant survey scores.

Next, we looked at the youngest infants directly to see if they had an unusually large decline. This would also support the proposal that younger infants have large changes because the mothers are inexperienced rather than because the frenotomy intervention helped. The five youngest children in the control group were selected with ages in days of 5, 8, 9, 17, and 19. The changes in survey scores of these children were 3, 0, 4, 25, and 24,respectively. Only two of the set showed a decline in survey scores. In other words, the youngest members of the control group (i.e., those members presumably the most comparable to the frenotomy group) displayed relatively little change in their survey scores. This is again the opposite of what we would expect to see if age was a key factor in explaining improvements in infant survey scores.

Although statistical analysis cannot remove the age-matching limitation of the current design, the analyses failed to support age as a meaningful factor influencing infant survey scores. Although the difference in age between the frenotomy and breastfeeding support infants did trend toward statistical significance, we saw no evidence that age actually influenced survey scores. Further analyses excluded age as a variable of interest.

Testing the Effect of Condition and Time on Survey Scores

The primary analysis focused on testing the hypothesis that the surgical intervention influenced tongue-tie survey scores. The means, standard deviations, and confidence intervals for the breastfeeding support and frenotomy groups—before and after the postsurgery time window—are summarized in Table 2.

A summary of individual trends is displayed in Figure 4 to contrast individual and group trends and to allow for identification of possible outliers. Figure 5 compares the mean trends—along with their 95% confidence intervals—directly to make it easier to visually examine the data for a possible condition by time interaction.

Table 2. Descriptive Statistics for Survey Scores by Condition and Time					
Condition	Time	n	Mean	SD	95% CI
Control	After	15	23.73	3.87	2.14
Control	Before	15	25.87	3.87	2.14
Frenotomy	After	20	20.60	6.51	3.05
Frenotomy	Before	20	36.75	6.51	3.05

Note. Standard deviation and confidence intervals calculated here make use of the shared variability within groups.

The condition by time interaction was tested formally using a mixed-methods 2 x 3 x 2 ANOVA with condition as a between-groups factor and time as a within-subjects factor, $F(33) = 27.34$, $p < .01$, $R^2 = 0.16$.

ANOVA is the conventional analysis for testing the effect of independent factors on an outcome variable—here the effect of group (frenotomy vs. breastfeeding support) and time (preintervention and postintervention) on survey scores. The results of this analysis suggest that whether or not the infant group had an effect on survey scores depends on which time we assess at. In other words, there was a significant interaction between group and time. In the presence of a significant interaction, the main effect—determined by testing for the effects of group and time alone—are often difficult or even nonsensical to interpret. In our analysis, they were ignored and t-tests were conducted to test for differences between the four condition-by-time cells (i.e., simple effects). These results are summarized in Table 3.

Table 3. Summary of Simple Effects Analyses			
Comparison	t Value	p Value	R^2
Control, before vs. control, after	1.51	.15	.14
Frenotomy, before vs. frenotomy, after	7.84	<.01	.76
Control, before vs. frenotomy, before	−4.54	<.01	.47
Control, after vs. frenotomy, after	1.31	.20	.06

Note. R^2 is provided as a measure of effect size.

Discussion

Mothers whose babies have ankyloglossia are thought to be at higher risk for breastfeeding symptoms. By convention, ankyloglossia is typically treated via lingual frenotomy. We set out in this article to first assess the effectiveness of lingual frenotomy on reducing breastfeeding symptoms, and second to begin exploring the extent to which infants diagnosed with ankyloglossia suffer more symptoms as compared to infants whose mothers simply sought out breastfeeding support.

Figure 4. Individual and Mean Trends in Survey Scores for Each Infant in the Two Study Conditions

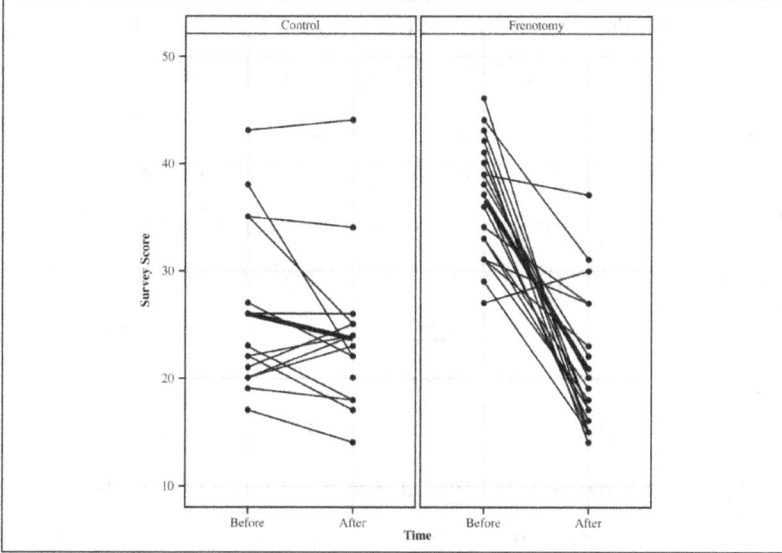

Each thin line represents the direction and steepness of change of one infant's survey scores between the first and second measurements. The thick lines represent the direction and steepness of change in each group's mean scores between the first and second measurements.

Figure 5. Line Plot of Group Mean Survey Scores

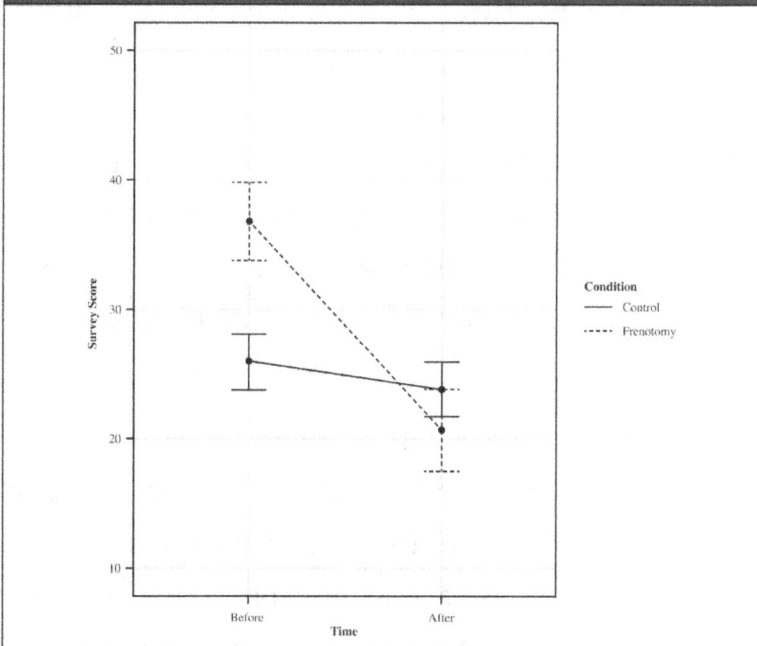

This takes the mean trends shown in Figure 4 and superimposes them over each other to aid in visualizing possible condition by time interactions. The whiskers represent the 95% confidence interval for each mean.

We hypothesized that infants having frenotomy should show a decline in survey scores, indicating a decrease in breastfeeding symptoms. Infants in the control condition—representing a baseline for survey scores mothers should report for nondiagnosed sources of breastfeeding symptoms—should change relatively little. Both data visualization and formal statistical analyses supported this hypothesis. The frenotomy-group data showed a significant decline in symptom severity after frenotomy. There was no evidence that the breastfeeding support groups showed a decline in scores between measurements—although these infants may have already benefited from the support group sessions and stabilized prior to the first survey administration.

Interestingly, there was no evidence that infants in the frenotomy group, and those in the breastfeeding support group, differed in their level of breastfeeding symptoms after the intervention. Caution is due when interpreting null results, but the overall patterning of the data is supportive of the conclusion that frenotomy is effective at reducing breastfeeding symptoms in infants with ankyloglossia.

In addition to serving as a subjective measure of breastfeeding symptoms, the Breastfeeding Symptom Survey was developed to help mothers recognize breast-feeding symptoms as early as possible and bring this to the attention of their lactation consultant or physician to determine the underlying cause of the symptoms.

This proposal, however, is dependent on there being a reasonably consistent relationship between an infant having ankyloglossia and having breastfeeding symptoms. Prior to the frenotomy intervention, the frenotomy group showed higher survey scores than the control group. This may suggest that infants with ankyloglossia have more breastfeeding symptoms than the baseline of infants with breastfeeding difficulties. However, the mother–infant pairs in the frenotomy group were self-selecting—they represent infants with ankyloglossia who are also experiencing breastfeeding symptoms. It is possible that there are at least some infants with ankyloglossia who breastfeed normally.

The extent to which ankyloglossia is a risk factor for breastfeeding symptoms has not been well studied. We have neither good estimate of how much more likely breastfeeding symptoms are as a result of having tongue-tie, nor how much more likely it is that an infant has ankyloglossia if she has breastfeeding symptoms. Measurements of breastfeeding symptoms, like the Breastfeeding Symptom Survey, will likely be useful in assessing this relationship and—if the relationship is reasonably strong—may serve as an early means of detecting babies at risk for a problematic case of tongue-tie. At the very least, such surveys help identify mothers who could benefit from some kind of assistance—be it from a lactation consultant, physician, or a breastfeeding support group—and they may assist physicians in determining whether a lingual frenotomy is merited (e.g., if a baby has ankyloglossia but no breastfeeding symptoms, intervention might be deferred).

There are important design limitations to keep in mind when considering these results. The lack of age matching means that age remains a viable alternative to the frenotomy intervention as an explanation for why survey scores declined. The mothers in our frenotomy group were largely self-selected—they were experiencing severe breastfeeding symptoms including immense pain and frustration—and so were highly motivated to seek help as quickly as possible. This may explain why the frenotomy group infants tend to be younger than the control group. It is possible that, if untreated, these infants would have improved naturally over time as their mothers gained more breastfeeding experience. Evidence from our analyses strongly suggests that this is not the case, and that age is not a confounding factor, but it should not be completely ruled out.

Another limitation is the samples were those of convenience and neither parents nor the practitioner were blinded. It would also be desirable to have ankyloglossia patients randomized to frenotomy or no frenotomy (or, better, a *sham* frenotomy or some alternative).

The difficulty of recruiting for and executing such a design, however, is high and was part of the motivation for the current design.

Overall, I propose two tentative conclusions based on this study results. First, the results support the use of lingual frenotomy as a reasonable intervention for infants who have ankyloglossia and are experiencing breast-feeding symptoms. Second, the results illustrate the use of the Breastfeeding Symptom Survey (freely available at http://babytonguetie.com/) for exploring links between tongue-tie and breastfeeding symptoms and—pending further work—as a possible means of early identification of infants who might benefit from medical intervention.

References

Amir, L. H., James, J. P., & Beatty, J. (2005). Review of tongue-tie release at a tertiary maternity hospital. *Journal of Paediatric and Child Health, 41*(5), 243–245.

Buryk, M., Bloom, D., & Shope, T. (2011). Efficacy of neonatal release of ankyloglossia: A randomized trial. *Pediatrics, 128*(2), 280–288.

Coryllos, E., Watson Genna, C., & Salloum, A. C. (2004, Summer). Congenital tongue-tie and its impact on breastfeeding. *Breastfeeding: Best for Baby and Mother*, pp. 1–2.

Dollberg, S., Botzer, E., Grunis, E., & Mimouni, F. B. (2006). Immediate nipple pain relief after frenotomy in breast-fed infants with ankyloglossia: A randomized, prospective study. *Journal of Pediatric Surgery, 41*, 1598–1600.

Edmunds, J. E., Fulbrook, P., & Miles, S. (2013). Understanding the experiences of mothers who are breastfeeding an infant with tongue-tie: A phenomenological study. *Journal of Human Lactation, 29*(2), 190–195.

Edmunds, J., Miles, S. C., & Fulbrook, P. (2011). Tongue-tie and breastfeeding: A review of the literature. *Breastfeeding Review, 19*(1), 19–26.

Griffiths, D. M. (2004). Do tongue ties affect breastfeeding? *Journal of Human Lactation, 20*, 409–414.

Hazelbaker, A. K. (2010). *Tongue-tie: Morphogenesis, impact, assessment and treatment*. Columbus, OH: Aidan and Eva Press.

Hogan, M., Westcott, C., & Griffiths, D. M. (2005). Randomized controlled division of tongue-tie infants with breastfeeding problems. *Journal of Paediatric & Child Health, 41*(5–6), 246–250.

Hong, P., Lago, D., Seargeant, J., Pellman, L., Magit, A. E., & Pransky, S. M. (2010). Defining ankyloglossia: A case series of anterior and posterior tongue ties. *International Journal of Pediatric Otorhinolaryngology, 74*, 1003–1006.

Miranda, B. H., & Milroy, C. J. (2010). A quick snip: A study of the impact of outpatient tongue-tie release on neonatal growth and breastfeeding. *Journal of Plastic, Reconstructive, & Aesthetic Surgery, 63*(9), e683–e685.

O'Callahan, C., Macary, S., & Clemente, S. (2013). The effects of office-based frenotomy for anterior and posterior ankyloglossia on breastfeeding. *International Journal of Pediatric Otorhinolaryngology, 77*(5), 827–832.

Acknowledgments: The author thanks Brian Waismeyer, MA; Gail Ecker, RN, IBCLC, RLC; and Fraser Cocks, PhD, for the time and expertise they each contributed to this project. The author also is indebted to Reviewers 1 and 2 for their helpful and constructive comments. This article as presented at the Society for Ear, Nose and Throat Advances in Children meeting on December 1, 2012, in Charleston, SC.

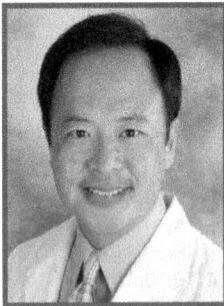

James W. Ochi, MD, is a fellowship-trained pediatric otolaryngologist board-certified in both otolaryngology and medical acupuncture. He provides integrative care to children with ear, nose, and throat problems. Dr. Ochi has a voluntary faculty appointment in the Department of Surgery at UC San Diego School of Medicine, and has been in private practice for more than 20 years in San Diego.

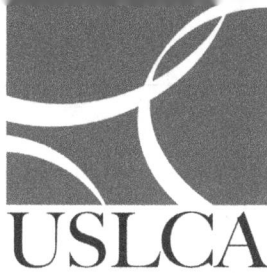

Early Frenotomy Improves Breastfeeding Outcomes for Tongue-Tied Infants

Asti Praborini, MD, IBCLC, RLC[1]

Hani Purnamasari, MD[2]

Agusnawati Munandar, MD, IBCLC, RLC[3]

Ratih Ayu Wulandari, MD, IBCLC, RLC[4]

Keywords: Breastfeeding, tongue-tie, frenotomy, lactogenesis

Although there is evidence to suggest that frenotomy improves breastfeeding outcomes for tongue-tied (ankyloglossic) infants, less is known about the optimal timing of treatment. In this retrospective cohort study, the timing of frenotomy and its impact on infant and maternal

1   astipraborini@yahoo.com
2   hani_purnamasari@yahoo.com
3   wati_arkan@yahoo.com
4   dr.ratih@menjadiibu.com

factors were examined in 31 tongue-tied babies with breastfeeding difficulties in a hospital in Jakarta, Indonesia. After frenotomy, all infants improved latching and mothers experienced a subjective improvement in nipple pain and breast engorgement. Frenotomy improved weight gain in infants regardless of type of tongue-tie (p < .001), but greater mean weight gains were achieved in tongue-tied babies who underwent early frenotomy (prior to Day 8) compared to babies who underwent late frenotomy (after Day 8; p < 0.002). Tongue-tie and frenotomy issues need to be addressed during the very first few days of an infant's life to ensure optimal breastfeeding outcomes.

The International Affiliation of Tongue-tie Professionals defines *tongue-tie* (ankyloglossia) as *an embryological remnant of tissue in the midline between the undersurface of the tongue and the floor of the mouth that restricts normal tongue movement* (International Affiliation of Tongue-tie Professionals, 2014).

The incidence of tongue-tie is reported to be between 1% and 10%, and its association with breastfeeding difficulties is well documented (Ballard, Auer, & Khoury, 2002; Messner, Lalakea, Aby, Macmahon, & Bair, 2000).

These problems include maternal nipple pain, slow infant weight gain, infant breast refusal, and low maternal milk supply because of poor milk removal (Garbin et al., 2013). Frenotomy, in which the lingual frenulum is cut, has been shown to effectively resolve breastfeeding difficulties caused by infants with tongue-tie in several clinical studies (Buryk, Bloom, & Shope, 2011; Geddes et al., 2008; Knox, 2010; Mayer, 2012). However, there have only been limited studies on tongue-tie in Indonesia, and there is little data and no universal guidelines to inform practitioners on the optimal timing of frenotomy (Garbin et al., 2013). There are many videos available online about tongue-tie and breastfeeding. Here is a playlist to get you started:

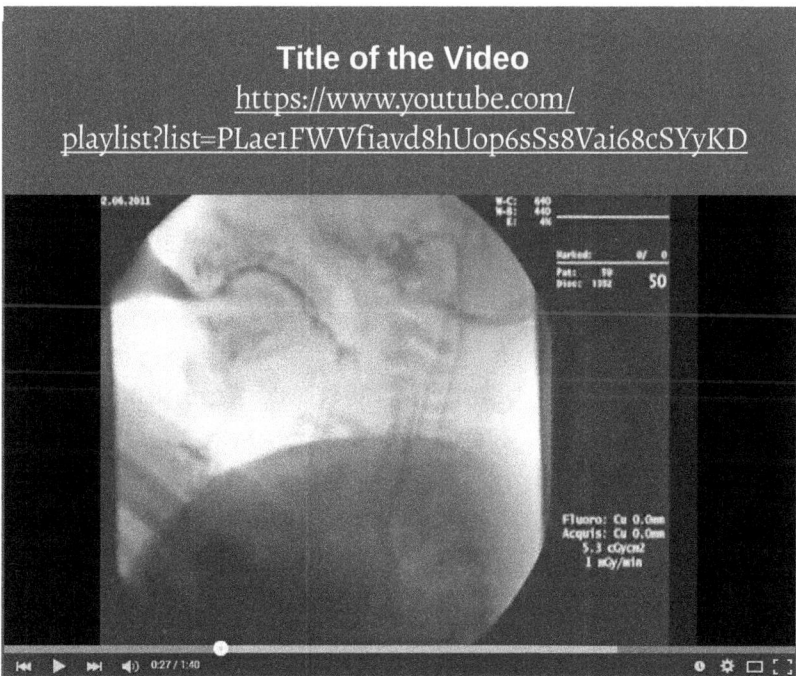

Title of the Video
https://www.youtube.com/
playlist?list=PLae1FWVfiavd8hUop6sSs8Vai68cSYyKD

We therefore examined the effects of early and late frenotomy on breastfeeding outcomes from the of both the mother and infant. We demonstrate that frenotomy performed as soon as possible, and ideally prior to Day 8, has a greater impact on improving weight gain compared to frenotomy performed after Day 8.

Method

Sample

All pediatric consultation files between January and June 2011 in a hospital with pediatric facilities in South Jakarta, Indonesia, were reviewed. There were 505 patient consultations over the study period, from which 62 tongue-tie cases were identified, for an overall incidence of 12.3% in our population; half of these were excluded because of loss to follow-up, leaving 31 cases available for study. Mothers and infants presented with various complaints: Mother complaints included sore nipple(s), breast engorgement, mastitis, pain during breastfeeding, and blocked ducts or nipple pores, whereas infant problems included latching only to the nipple, having a long period of breastfeeding without satiety, rage during breastfeeding, excessive weight loss, or not achieving the recommended weight gain. The subjects' characteristics are shown in Table 1.

A thorough history and examination was performed in all cases, including examination of the mother's breast, breastfeeding dyad, and baby's mouth. Where tongue-tie was found, it was observed to significantly interfere with the breastfeeding dyad. Babies were subsequently grouped according to the Coryllos classification of ankyloglossia, as shown in Table 2 (Genna, 2013).

Babies' weights were plotted using the World Health Organization (WHO) Anthro growth and development software. Growth was classified as *good* if the weight

Table 1. Characteristics of Study Subjects	
Characteristics	N = 31 (%)
Gender	
Male	13 (42%)
Female	18 (58%)
Age	
0–30 days	17 (55%)
1–6 months	14 (45%)
Tongue-tie type	
1	3 (10%)
2	10 (32%)
3	12 (38%)
4	6 (20%)
Age when frenotomy was done	
0–8 days	8 (26%)
>8 days	23 (74%)
Frenotomy indication	
Mother's complain	7 (22%)
Baby's complain	7 (22%)
Mother + baby complain	17 (56%)
Nutritional status	
Failure to thrive	13 (42%)
• An infant with body weight under the 3rd percentile or Z score < − 2. This occurred when the infant continued to lose weight after the age of 10 days and did not return to their birth weight by the age of 3 weeks or remained below the 10th percentile by the end of the first month of life.	
Slow weight gain	10 (32%)
• An infant less than 2 weeks of age who is more than 10% less than the birth weight or who is 2 weeks to 3 months of age whose weight gain is less than 20 g/day	
Well growth	8 (26%)
• An infant whose weight increases according to the World Health Organization exclusively breastfed growth curves	

increased according to the growth curve (Ng, 2010), whereas weight gain was classified as *slow* if infants less than 2 weeks of age had weight 10% less than the birth weight or infants 2 weeks to 3 months of age gained less than 20 g/day (Walker, 2011a).

Failure to thrive was defined as body weight under the 3rd percentile or Z score ,< - 2, which occurred if the baby continued to lose weight after 10 days and did not return to their birth weight by 3 weeks, or were below the 10th percentile at the end of the first month of life (Ng, 2010).

Table 2. Coryllos Classification of Ankyloglossia

Type	Superior Attachment	Inferior Attachment	Characteristic of Frenulum
1	Tip of tongue	Alveolar ridge	Often thin, may be elastic
2	2–4 mm behind tongue tip	On or just behind alveolar ridge	Often thin, may be elastic
3	Mid tongue	Middle of floor of mouth	Usually thicker, more fibrous, inelastic
4	Submucosal	Floor of mouth at base of tongue	Usually thick, fibrous, shiny, and inelastic

Source: Genna, C. W. (2013). *Supporting sucking skills in breastfeeding infants.* Sudbury, MA: Jones and Bartlett.

Classification of Frenotomy

Babies were also grouped by the timing of the frenotomy, early and late, which we refer to lactogenesis stage. Lactogenesis Stage II marks the onset of copious milk secretion between Day 3–8; milk synthesis occurs even in the absence of infant suckling or milk expression. Lactogenesis Stage III (Day 9 to the beginning of involution) is the maintenance of established milk production via autocrine control (Riordan, 2010).

Although lactogenesis Stages II and III are physiologic processes, and cannot be defined by days of age, for the purposes of this retrospective chart review, we are using days of age as a proxy for stage of lactogenesis, *early frenotomy* refer to babies who underwent frenotomy in between Day 3 and 8, and *late frenotomy* refer to babies who underwent frenotomy after Day 9.

Procedure

Parents received a full explanation about tongue-tie and frenotomy and gave written informed consent prior to the procedure. In preparation for frenotomy, the baby was swaddled to immobilize the arms and legs and laid supine on the examination table. An assistant helped by holding the head still while the operator lifted the tongue with a finger to locate the problematic frenulum. The area was disinfected by applying povidone-iodine with swab sticks, as described previously (Sunil Kumar, Raja Babu, Jagadish Reddy, & Uttam, 2011).

The frenulum was then snipped with blunt-ended sterile scissors, and sterile gauze was used to attain hemostasis. The tongue-tie was assessed as completely released if a neat diamond shape was visible with no palpable tissue remaining to restrict tongue movement. We favored not using general anesthesia to perform the procedure because this is likely to add delays in breastfeeding.

Immediately after frenotomy, the mother was asked to breastfeed her baby for reevaluation of latch and improvement. The mother was taught how to perform tongue exercises to prevent reattachment, and a review was scheduled 3 days later to assess for complications and evaluate weight gain. A further review was scheduled 1 week later and continued every week thereafter as necessary until the breastfeeding dyads' course was deemed satisfactory.

Data Collection and Analyses

Weight loss data were collected by comparing weight at the time of frenotomy to that infant's birth weight and dividing that by the age of the baby in days on the day of frenotomy. Weight gain data were collected by comparing weight upon the baby review and dividing days on the day of frenotomy. The review time was between 3 days to 1 week after frenotomy.

Standard WHO growth data show that even infants born at and following the 1st percentile gain, at minimum, 30 g/day. However, the WHO system has been shown to result in false positives for the *underweight* category in some breastfed infants during the first 6 months, resulting in unnecessary supplementation or early use of complementary foods (Walker, 2014). Therefore, we regarded a minimum weight gain per day of 20 g to be satisfactory (Ng, 2010).

Data were analyzed using SPSS Version 19. The paired t-test was performed to analyze differences in mean weight gain before and after frenotomy. Differences in absolute weight gain before and after frenotomy according to lactogenesis stages were analyzed using the Wilcoxon test.

Results

None of the babies had a good latch prior to frenotomy, in spite of otherwise good breastfeeding positions. Babies nibbled the nipple, made clicking sounds, had dimpled cheeks during breastfeeding, or retracted their lower lip during sucking. After frenotomy, all babies improved their latch. No serious side effects were observed after frenotomy: 6 (20%) babies had minor bleeding that stopped soon after breastfeeding, and at 3 days post-frenotomy, 28 (90%) babies had no observable complications.

A white, diamond-shaped wound was observed in three (10%) subjects that disappeared on follow-up a week later. Subjectively, mothers experienced immediate relief after frenotomy, with 27 mothers reporting improvement in nipple pain and breast engorgement after one week, with the remainder improving by two weeks.

The weight loss and gain differences before and after frenotomy for each type of tongue-tie are shown in Table 3.

The type of tongue-tie was not associated with weight gain or weight loss. The mean differences in weight loss and weight gain (in grams per day) before and after frenotomy according to type of tongue-tie are shown in Figure 1.

Regardless of tongue-tie type, the mean weight loss prior to frenotomy was 18.52 g/day, and the mean weight gain after frenotomy was 27.65 g/day, which was significantly different (p = .001).

Furthermore, babies lost an average of 65 g/day in weight prior to frenotomy and increased their weight by an average of 38 g/day after frenotomy at lactogenesis Stage II (p < .002), whereas lactogenesis Stage III babies gained an average of 5 g/day prior to frenotomy, but gained 20 g/day after frenotomy, although this change was not statistically significant (p < .170; see Figure 2).

Discussion

Here, we examined the effect of frenotomy on infant weight gain from the perspectives of both the infants and mothers. Frenotomy resulted in significant improvements in weight gain in infants, which was more marked if the frenotomy was performed before Day 8. Since this time point is likely to correspond to lactogenesis Stage II, we hypothesize that optimizing breastfeeding by frenotomy in tongue-tied infants at the same time as the onset of copious milk production contributes to improved early outcomes, at least in terms of weight gain.

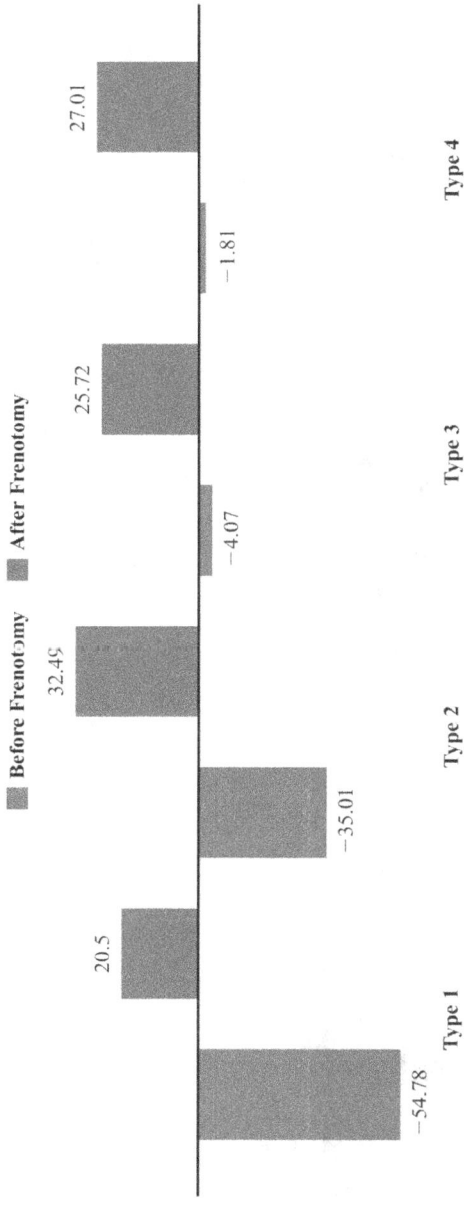

Figure 1. Mean Differences in Weight Loss and Weight Gain Before and After Frenotomy on Each Type of Tongue-Tie (g/day)

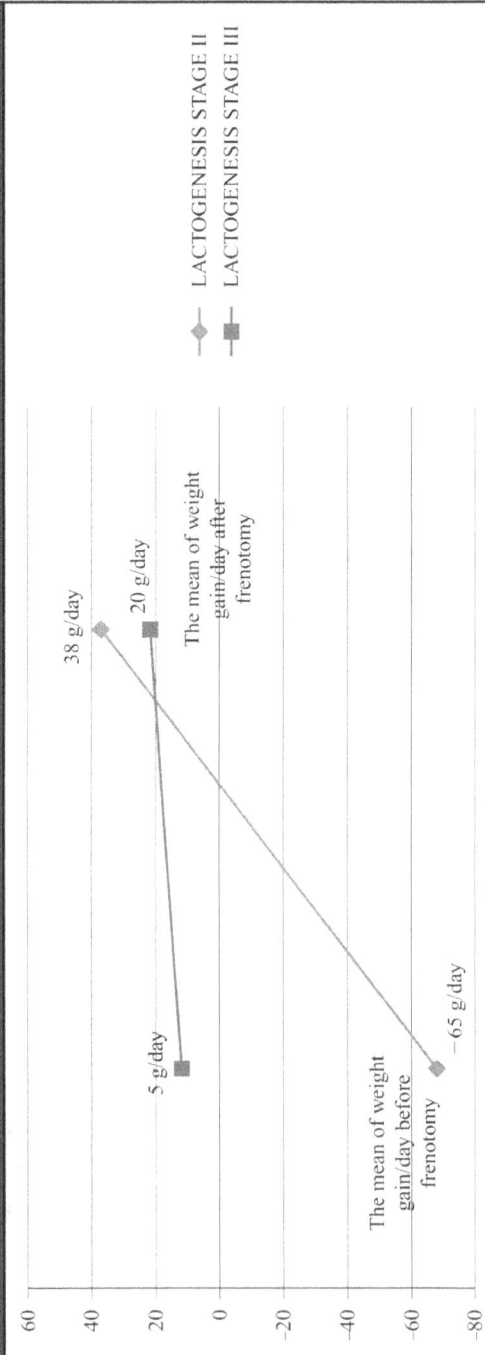

Figure 2. Comparison of Weight Gain Before and After Frenotomy Based on Lactogenesis Stage

Table 3. Weight Loss and Weight Gain Differences Before and After Frenotomy on Each Type of Tongue-Tie

Difference in Weight (g/day)	Tongue-Tie Type			
	Type 1 (N = 3)	Type 2 (N = 10)	Type 3 (N = 12)	Type 4 (N = 6)
The mean of weight loss before frenotomy	54.78	35.01	4.07	1.81
The mean of weight gain after frenotomy	20.50	32.49	25.72	27.01
Greatest weight loss	35	150	155	33
Greatest weight gain	185	152	45	42

This finding is in line with a retrospective study by (Steehler, Steehler, & Harley, 2012), who examined data on 367 tongue-tied infants with breastfeeding problems seen over a 5-year period. Based on subjective maternal observations, frenotomy performed on neonates with ankyloglossia and feeding difficulties in the first week of life exhibited more benefit than those who received the procedure after the first week of life.

To ensure successful breastfeeding, health workers who help mothers to breastfeed need to be aware of the complexity and importance of coordinated tongue movements by the infant during feeding.

For successful milk extraction, the tongue needs to perform several actions. First, the tongue extends over the lower gum to inhibit the bite reflex and contribute to an airtight seal on the areola to create an intraoral vacuum and promote milk flow from the breast. Second, the tongue needs to manipulate the nipple and areolar tissue into a proper relationship with the hard and soft palates, the tongue itself, and the swallowing/breathing apparatus. Limitation of the tongue's free movement leads to suboptimal nursing mechanics.

The nipple's spatial relationship to the infant's mouth structures and the specific pattern of tongue movements are critical both for effective and efficient milk removal and to protect the delicate nipple tissue from trauma. The harmful effects of tongue-tie are either related to ineffective breast emptying, to nipple trauma, or both (Knox, 2010).

Here, we compared two groups: early frenotomy (prior to Day 8 and equivalent to lactogenesis Stage II) and late frenotomy (after Day 8 and equivalent to lactogenesis Stage III).

Lactogenesis refers to the transition from pregnancy to lactation. Lactogenesis Stage I occurs from mid-pregnancy to postpartum Day 2, lactogenesis Stage II from Day 3–8, and lactogenesis Stage III starts on Day 9 and continues to the beginning of involution (Riordan, 2010). After birth, following placental delivery, progesterone levels decline rapidly, resulting in increased prolactin levels and triggering the start of lactogenesis Stage II and the onset of copious milk secretion. Milk synthesis occurs during lactogenesis Stage II even in the absence of infant suckling or milk expression. The volume of milk production increases from 37 ml on Day 1 to 408 ml on Day 3 (the beginning of lactogenesis Stage II), whereas milk volume continues to increase to 576 ml on Day 7 and averages 750 ml by 4 weeks (Walker, 2010b).

Lactogenesis Stage III, also known as *galactopoiesis,* is the maintenance of the established milk production via autocrine (local) control, in which one type of cell in the gland regulates adjacent cells in the same gland.

Frequent and complete milk removal by feeding is proposed to enhance milk production by removing breast milk constituents that exert negative feedback on breast secretory cells. In this way, removal of milk by the infant controls synthesis and is referred to as the *supply-versus-demand response* (Black, Jarman, & Simpson, 1998).

Although suckling (or mechanical milk removal) may not be a prerequisite for lactogenesis Stage II, it is critical for lactogenesis Stage III. However, the quantity and quality of infant suckling or milk removal governs breast milk synthesis (Riordan, 2010).

Geddes et al. (2008) identified two irregular tongue movements that occur in tongue-tied babies during breastfeeding, which result in compression of the base or the tip of the nipple and may contribute to maternal pain, decreased milk transfer, and consequent slowing weight gain and failure to thrive.

Using ultrasound, the same group also showed that frenotomy can resolve irregular tongue movements and improve milk intake, milk transfer rate, attachment to the breast, and maternal pain. Babies undergoing early frenotomy not only nursed at the breast effectively and efficiently, improving both milk transfer and milk production, but also had sufficient milk volume from intrinsic Stage II milk production to significantly increase weight in these babies. However, late frenotomy (after Day 8), while improving the babies' latch, only resulted in small increases in weight. This is likely to be because of the late release of the tongue-tie creating only a low demand response, leading to low milk transfer and insufficient milk production. Mothers experienced low milk supply, resulting in only small weight gains in these babies who were only breastfed.

Our study was limited by being a retrospective review of medical records, with some records being incomplete. In addition, no control comparison was made with infants not undergoing frenotomy. Further prospective studies with larger sample sizes are required.

Conclusion

For successful lactation, identification of tongue-tie at birth and close monitoring of feeding may help to detect milk-supply problems sooner. Frenotomy is an effective, simple, and safe treatment for tongue-tied babies experiencing breastfeeding difficulties. Early frenotomy, prior to Day 8, appears to have a larger impact on weight gain and lactation performance, hence leading to more successful breastfeeding outcomes.

References

Ballard, J. L., Auer, C. E., & Khoury, J. C. (2002). Ankyloglossia: Assessment, incidence, and effect of frenuloplasty on the breastfeeding dyad. *Pediatrics, 110*(5), 63. Retrieved from http://www.pediatrics.org/cgi/content/full/110/5/e63

Black, R. F., Jarman, L., & Simpson, J. B. (1998). *The science of breastfeeding* (Vol. 3). Ontario, Canada: Jones and Bartlett.

Buryk, M., Bloom, D., & Shope, T. (2011). Efficacy of neonatal release of ankyloglossia: A randomized trial. *Pediatrics, 128*(2), 280–288.

Garbin, C. P., Sakalidis, V. S.,Chadwick, L. M., Whan, E., Hartmann, P. E., & Geddes, D. T. (2013). Evidence of improved milk intake after frenotomy: A case report. *Pediatrics, 132*(5), e1413–e1417.

Geddes, D. T., Langton, D. B., Gollow, I., Jacobs, L. A., Hartmann, P. E., & Simmer, K. (2008). Frenulotomy for breastfeeding infants with ankyloglossia: Effect on milk removal and sucking mechanism as imaged by ultrasound. *Pediatrics, 122*, e188–e194.

Genna, C. W. (2013). *Supporting sucking skills in breastfeeding infants.* Sudbury, MA: Jones and Bartlett. International Affiliation of Tongue-tie Professionals. (2014). *Definition of tongue-tie.* Retrieved from http://tonguetieprofessionals.org/about/assessment/definition-of-tongue-tie/

Knox, I. (2010). Tongue tie and frenotomy in the breastfeeding newborn. *Neoreviews*, *11*(9), e513–e519. Retrieved from http://neoreviews.aappublications.org/content/11/9/e513.short

Mayer, D. R. (2012, January 1). Frenotomy for breastfed tongue-tied infants: A fresh look at an old procedure. *AAP News*, *33*, 12.

Messner, A. H., Lalakea, M. L., Aby, J., Macmahon, J., & Bair, E. (2000). Ankyloglossia: Incidence and associated feeding difficulties. *Archives of Otolaryngology—Head and Neck Surgery*, *126*(1), 36–39.

Ng, P. (2010). Low intake in the breastfeeding infant: Maternal and infant considerations. In J. Riordan & K. Wambach (Eds.), *Breastfeeding and human lactation* (4th ed., pp. 325–363). Sudbury, MA: Jones and Bartlett.

Riordan, J. (2010). Anatomical and biological imperatives. In J. Riordan & K. Wambach (Eds.), *Breastfeeding and human lactation* (4th ed., pp. 77–112). Sudbury, MA: Jones and Bartlett.

Steehler, M. W., Steehler, M. K., & Harley, E. H. (2012). A retrospective review of frenotomy in neonates and infants with feeding difficulties. *International Journal of Pediatric Otorhinolaryngology*, *76*(9), 1236–1240.

Sunil Kumar, P., Raja Babu, P., Jagadish Reddy, G., & Uttam, A. (2011). Povidone iodine—Revisited. *Indian Journal of Dental Advancements*, *3*(3), 617–620.

Walker, M. (2011a). Beyond the initial 48–72 hours: Infant challenges. In *Breastfeeding management for the clinician: Using the evidence* (2nd ed., pp. 347–427). Sudbury, MA: Jones and Bartlett.

Walker, M. (2011b). Influence of the maternal anatomy and physiology. In *Breastfeeding management for the clinician: Using the evidence* (2nd ed., pp. 75–131). Sudbury, MA: Jones and Bartlett.

Walker, M. (2014). Beyond the initial 48–72 hours: Infant challenges. In *Breastfeeding management for the clinician: Using the evidence* (3rd. ed., pp. 337–408). Burlington, MA: Jones and Bartlett.

Acknowledgments:

The authors would like to thank the Board of Directors of Kemang Medical Care Mother and Child Hospital for the permission and support, and also to Arisma and Pica from Indonesia Breastfeeding Association for their help and support.

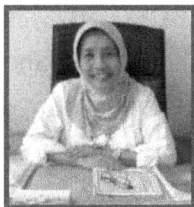

Asti Praborini, MD, Pediatrician, IBCLC, RLC, is a granny of a successful breastfeeding mother. Having 24 years of experience as a pediatrician convinced her that nothing is more important and valuable than breastfeeding for both mother and baby. As a national speaker, she continues to campaign for the benefit of breastfeeding despite the abundance of formula marketing. She built the first hospital-based lactation team in Indonesia that works ultimately to help mother breastfeed her baby. She is practicing frenotomy for anterior as well as posterior tongue-tie and lip-tie, established her method for hospitalization of nipple confusion, supplementation, adoptive nursing, and many others.

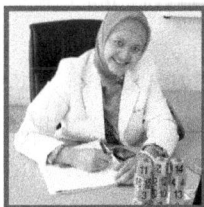

Hani Purnamasari, MD, Pediatrician, devoted her time in the lactation field after she found many babies had excessive weight loss and failure to thrive because of breastfeeding difficulties. She is joining the lactation team and now helping many mothers to achieve their breastfeeding goals. She is practicing frenotomy for anterior as well as posterior tongue-tie and lip-tie. Dr. Hani often speaks to promote the benefit of breastfeeding, and her best experience was sharing the same stage with Dr. Jack Newman (pediatrician) at the Seminar and Workshop of Breastfeeding Update on Daily Practice, in Jakarta, Indonesia.

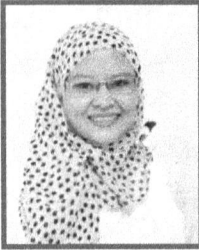

Agusnawati Munandar, MD, IBCLC, RLC, is a successful breastfeeding mother of two. She decided to enter the lactation field because she wants to embrace breastfeeding and help many mothers to succeed. She is working in a lactation clinic of baby-friendly hospitals and earned her IBCLC degree in 2013. She is involved in a lactation team that helps many mothers to achieve their breastfeeding goals, such as practicing frenotomy for anterior as well as posterior tongue-tie and lip-tie, hospitalization for nipple confusion, supplementation, adoptive nursing, and others.

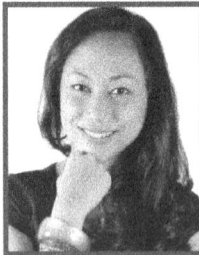

Ratih Ayu Wulandari, MD, IBCLC, RLC, entered the lactation field once she realized that breastfeeding mothers need help and support. Having experienced breastfeeding her tongue-tied baby helps her understand the pain and to support early frenotomy. She is now joining the lactation team and practicing frenotomy for anterior as well as posterior tongue-tie and lip-tie. She believes attachment parenting is the best way to nurture a child and shares her thoughts on her blog http://www.menjadiibu.com.

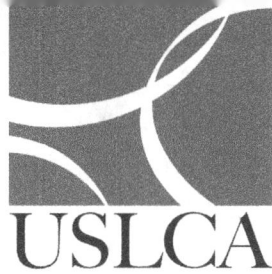

Does Kinesio Elastic Therapeutic Taping Decrease Breast Engorgement in Postpartum Women?

Donna Brown, RN, IBCLC, RLC[1]
Claire Langdon, MA, RN, IBCLC, RLC[2]

Keywords: Engorgement, Kinesio taping

Breast engorgement is a common problem in the early postpartum period. The purpose of this study was to determine the effectiveness of Kinesio Elastic Therapeutic Taping® (K-ETT), used to increase lymphatic drainage or decrease fluid in congested areas, in treating breast engorgement in postpartum women. Thirty-four healthy mothers who delivered healthy babies over a 4-week period in a large community hospital participated, with one

1   Lactation Services, El Camino Hospital, donna_brown@elcaminohospital.org,
2   Lactation Services, El Camino Hospital

breast taped and the other remaining untaped. Two subjective measures, self-reported pain and self-rated engorgement, and one objective measure, firmness by durometer measured by the researchers, were taken at baseline and throughout the study period. Engorgement was defined as exceeding a threshold in at least two of the three measures. Overall, 65% of mothers experienced engorgement. There was no difference in the incidence of engorgement, comparing the taped to the untaped breast by paired analysis. Future work in this area should include development and testing of valid and reliable measures of engorgement, followed by testing of interventions using a rigorous protocol to provide evidence for practice change.

Postpartum breast engorgement is a physiological condition that commonly occurs between days 3 and 5 postpartum and is characterized by a sudden increase in milk volume, lymphatic and vascular congestion, and interstitial edema (Hill & Humenick, 1994). Newton and Newton (1951) suggested that areolar distension from milk then led to compression of surrounding ducts, which subsequently led to secondary vascular and lymphatic compression (Academy of Breastfeeding Medicine [ABM] Protocol Committee, 2009). Engorgement has been estimated to occur in 20%–85% of mothers, based on numerous definitions and measures (Hill & Humenick, 1994). Postpartum breast engorgement can be a significant source of pain and breastfeeding difficulty (Stamp

& Casanove, 2006). Engorgement is occasionally so severe that, if left unresolved, it can lead to an inability to attach the baby for breastfeeding and loss of maternal milk supply (ABM, 2009).

Currently, the literature is limited regarding the prevention and effective treatment of postpartum breast engorgement (Mangesi & Dowswell, 2010). Frequent effective breastfeeding, softening at least one breast well per feeding, and alternating which breast is offered first, and breast massage after feeds are generally recognized as best practices for the prevention and treatment of engorgement. However, even with these measures, up to two thirds of postpartum women will experience at least moderate symptoms of engorgement (ABM, 2009).

One method recognized as effective (ABM, 2009; Riordan & Wambach, 2010) is reverse pressure softening (RPS), which is areolar massage that physically decreases edema of the areola to allow the infant to better attach and breastfeed (Cotterman, 2004). Current standard of practice also includes offering ice packs to engorged mothers for pain relief and to decrease breast swelling. A supportive bra and compression are sometimes recommended (Riordan & Wambach, 2010). Manual lymphatic massage has been reported as a successful treatment for postpartum breast engorgement (Chikly, 1999). Massage, cold, and compression are all accepted techniques used to decrease edema.

Kinesio Elastic Therapeutic Taping® (K-ETT) was invented in the 1970s by Kenzo Kase, DC (Kinesio Tex

Tape™) to reduce edema and increase lymphatic flow in joint injuries, primarily among athletes (http://www. kinesiotaping.com).

Several studies have examined the effectiveness of K-ETT in this setting (Shim, Lee, & Lee, 2003; Thelen, Dauber, & Stoneman, 2008; Tsai, Hung, Yang, Huang, & Tsauo, 2009; Yoshida & Kahanov, 2007). Shim et al. (2003) documented increased lymphatic flow after the use of K-ETT in animals.

Only one study has been conducted related to breast care; Tsai et al. (2009) demonstrated K-ETT to be equally effective as the current standard treatment of decongestive lymphatic therapy combined with pneumatic compression (Koul et al.,2007) in managing breast cancer–related lymphedema.

K-ETT differs from traditional tape in allowing full range of motion of the taped area, being lightweight and comfortable to wear over a 3–5-day period, being made from water-resistant cotton that wicks away moisture and allows the wearer to bathe as usual, and being latex-free so it is hypoallergenic (Kase & Stockheimer, 2006).

The purpose of our study was to investigate whether K-ETT has an effect on breast engorgement in breastfeeding mothers during the immediate postpartum period. We hypothesized that breastfeeding mothers would experience a decrease in breast engorgement by using the K-ETT method.

Method

Design and Sample

The design for this study was quasi-experimental and comparative. El Camino Hospital's Institutional Review Board approved the protocol. All healthy postpartum women on the maternity unit at El Camino Hospital aged 18–45 years who delivered a healthy baby, 38–41 weeks gestation, and with infant weighing more than 2,500 g were approached during a 4-week period.

Any mothers who were cognitively, visually, or physically impaired; who had language or hearing difficulties; or who had had previous breast surgery were eliminated as potential subjects. Mothers with fetal demise, or with babies in the neonatal intensive care unit (NICU), were not included in the study.

Procedure

Potential subjects were identified within 12–24 hours of delivery on the maternity unit at El Camino Hospital. The primary investigator explained the purpose of study, type, and length of subject involvement and potential risks; obtained written consent; and then applied a 2-inch piece of Kinesio® tape (hereafter called tape) to one breast as a test strip. The following day, Day 2 of the study, the primary investigator reconfirmed participant's willingness to continue in the study, answered any questions, and checked for any reaction to the tape. If there was no reaction to the tape, the primary investigator then took baseline measurements of breast pain, breast self-rated engorgement, and breast firmness, as well as demographic characteristics. She then applied tape to one breast (patient's choice), leaving the other breast untaped. Measurements of pain, self-rated engorgement, and breast firmness were repeated daily while mothers were in the hospital, with instructions given on how to self-measure and record pain and engorgement once discharged home.

Mothers were asked to return for breast firmness measurement on postpartum days 3 and 6. At the end of the study, anyone still wearing tape was asked to come to the hospital to have tape removed or given phone instructions on how to remove the tape at home.

The primary investigator, certified in the use of the tape, applied and monitored outcomes for all subjects. Application of tape included:

a) skin clean and dry, free of lotions;

b) two pieces of tape for each breast, 7–9 inches each, each piece further cut into five equal strips with an anchoring base and rounded corners (Figure 1);

c) avoiding the axilla, tape applied to breast with minimal stretch (10%–15% of which is tape off, no extra tension applied) leaving space around nipple/areola for infant to latch, tape ends not overlapping (Figure 2);

d) tape adhesive activated by patting and assessed for comfort and range of motion;

e) mother or investigator removed tape within 5 days.

A copy of the patient handout is available by request.

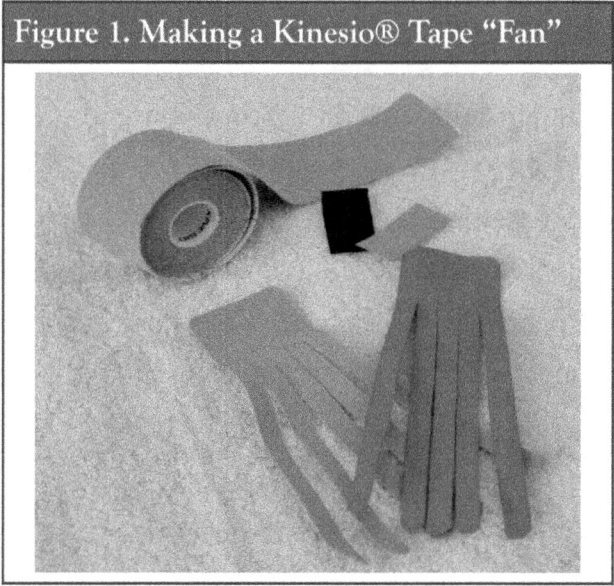

Figure 1. Making a Kinesio® Tape "Fan"

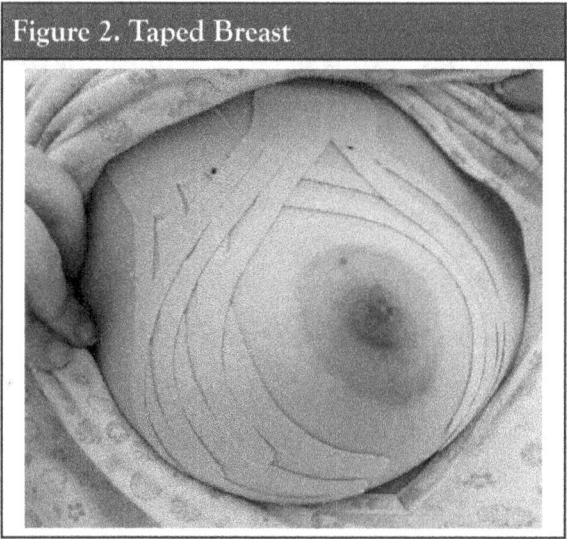

Figure 2. Taped Breast

Measures

The independent variable for this study was tape, with each mother serving as her own control, with one breast taped and the other remaining untaped.

The dependent variable was engorgement, using a combination of the following measures to ascertain whether engorgement was present or absent: Two subjective measures were pain and self-rated engorgement, and one objective measure was firmness. These measures were obtained separately for the taped and untaped breasts at baseline and over the course of the study.

Pain

Pain was assessed subjectively using the Bourbonnais pain scale (Figure 3), a subjective measure of self-rated pain on a numeric scale of 1–10 (10 being the worst possible pain; Bourbonnais, 1981). The threshold for pain was having at least one subsequent pain measure 3 points or more above baseline.

Self-Rated Engorgement

Self-rated engorgement was assessed using a scale (Figure 4) from 1 to 6 (1 being *soft, no change* and 6 being *very firm, very tender*; Hill & Humenick, 1994). Any measure of 3 (*firm, non-tender*) or more after baseline was the threshold for this subjective rating.

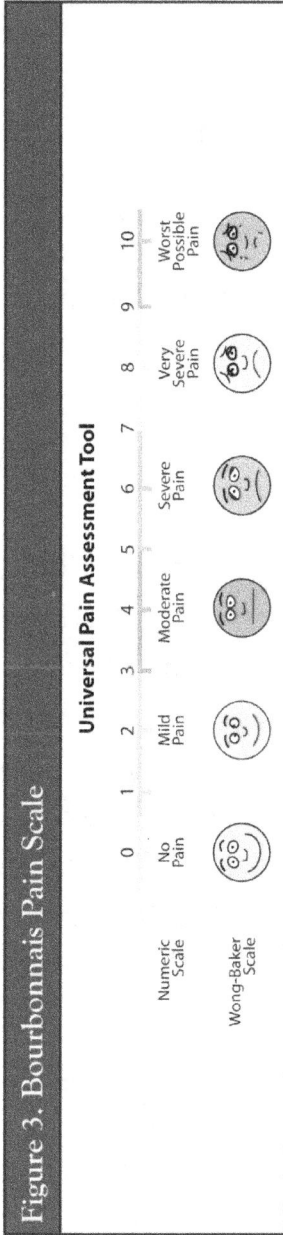

Figure 3. Bourbonnais Pain Scale

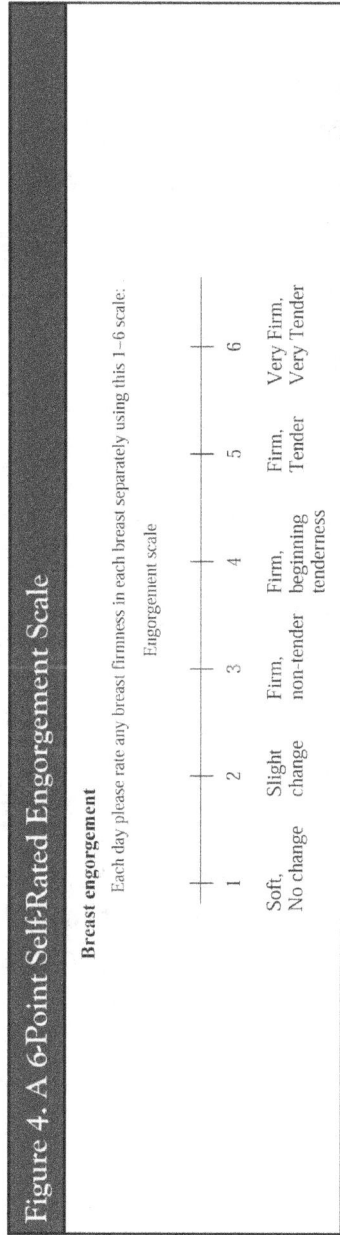

Figure 4. A 6-Point Self-Rated Engorgement Scale

Firmness

Breast firmness was objectively assessed by the investigator using a force gauge measuring how much force it takes to press a 75-mm plastic disc a set distance of 2.5 cm into an area of the breast, with measurements in pounds of force (Figure 5; Roberts, 1999).

A durometer is a force gauge used to measure hardness of a material, in this case, the breast. We used an IMADA brand, model no. DPS-11. The tip was custom-made to simulate size of fingertip pressing on skin, as one would do to palpate for edema.

One researcher obtained all the force gauge readings with one area of each breast marked and used for all subsequent measurements to minimize sampling variation (Roberts, 1999). Three readings were made and an average taken for each data point. Using the variation in the three force gauge readings averaged for each data point ($M = .0933$, SD $= .051$), and the fluctuations in force gauge readings for mothers with minimal breast changes during the 7 days of the study ($M = .148$, SD $= .076$), a difference in force gauge values of less than .20 was considered possible sampling variability.

The threshold for firmness was having the average of any subsequent reading at least .20 points higher than the average at baseline.

Mothers were asked to continue pain and self-rated engorgement measurements daily for both breasts at the same time of day, at maternal convenience, irrespective of breastfeeding times, for 3–6 days. Breast firmness was measured by the primary investigator on postpartum days 3 and 6.

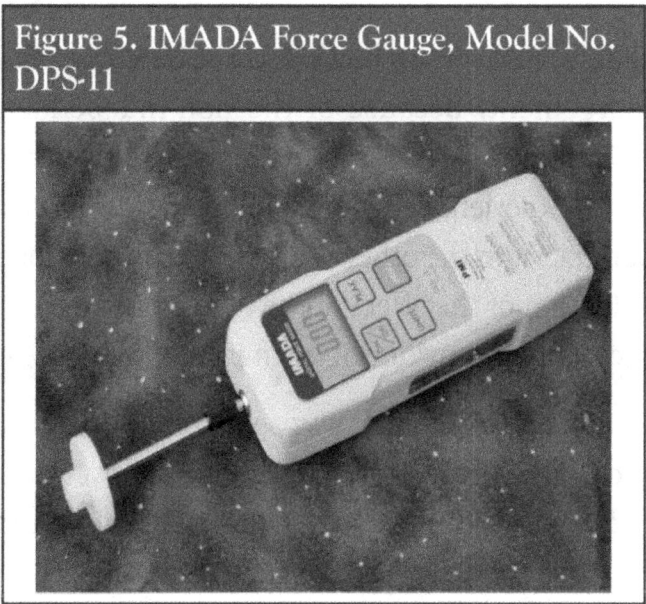

Figure 5. IMADA Force Gauge, Model No. DPS-11

Data Management and Analysis

Because the measures comprising the dependent variable of interest (engorgement) were subjective and objective, we determined that engorgement would be counted when at least two of the three measures exceeded the threshold.

This resulted in three dichotomous outcome measures when thresholds were exceeded: pain plus firmness, self-rated engorgement plus firmness, or pain plus self-rated engorgement. We were particularly interested in the first two measures because they represented the combination of one subjective measure and the objective measure, but we examined all three pairwise combinations. Mothers who had none or only one of the three measures exceeding the threshold were considered not to be engorged.

We conducted a paired analysis using McNemar's test (Glantz, 1997) on each of the three outcome measures of engorgement. Because of the non-independence of women's breasts—that is, a woman who was likely to perceive or experience engorgement in one breast was likely to experience it in the other—a paired analysis allowed for the evaluation of the effect of the tape on the incidence of engorgement by considering each *pair* of breasts.

For all analyses, alpha was set at .05 for determining statistical significance. We calculated the overall rate of engorgement as the number who had engorgement in either breast divided by the sample total, as well as rates according to the three outcomes defined earlier.

Results

Out of 318 deliveries during the 4-week study period, 214 mothers fit the study criteria and 64 initially provided informed consent and had tape placed to test for irritation.

On Day 2, 12 mothers opted out of the study for personal reasons, and 3 mothers dropped out because of itching from the tape. Of the 49 who continued, 20 chose to have the left breast taped and 29 chose the right.

After discharge from the hospital, the mothers had to come back to the hospital to complete measurements. This is where we lost 15 more mothers, leaving us with 34 mothers who had data on at least two measures between 4 and 7 days postpartum (Figure 6). The 34 mothers were from four ethnic groups: 47% White, 29% Southeast Asian (Indian), 15% Chinese, and 9% Other Asians. All 34 were married with college degrees, with an average age of 32 years, ranging from 27 to 40 years. Of those 23 of 34, 68% were first-time mothers, 8 were second-time mothers, and 3 were third-time mothers.

All who had a previous child or children had breastfed each for at least 6 weeks. Deliveries were vaginal (65%) or cesarean section (35%). All babies were term (38–41 weeks gestation), with an average birth weight of 7 lbs 7.4 oz, ranging from 5 lbs 13 oz to 8 lbs 11 oz, and 50% were boys, whereas 50% were girls.

The results of the McNemar's test, shown on Table 1, focus on mothers whose breasts differed in terms of being engorged or not.

Our results revealed that none of the definitions of engorgement, the two combinations of one subjective and the objective measure or the combination of the two subjective measures, showed differences in the incidence of engorgement between the taped and untaped breasts. For engorgement by pain and firmness, there was no difference in the taped versus untaped breasts ($p = 1.00$).

For engorgement by self-rated engorgement and firmness, there was also no significant difference seen between taped and untapped breasts in the paired analysis ($p = .375$). And likewise, for engorgement by pain and self-rated engorgement, the two subjective measures, there was no difference between taped versus untaped breasts (p = .375). Table 2 shows the breakdown of participants by whether they were engorged and the values of the measures.

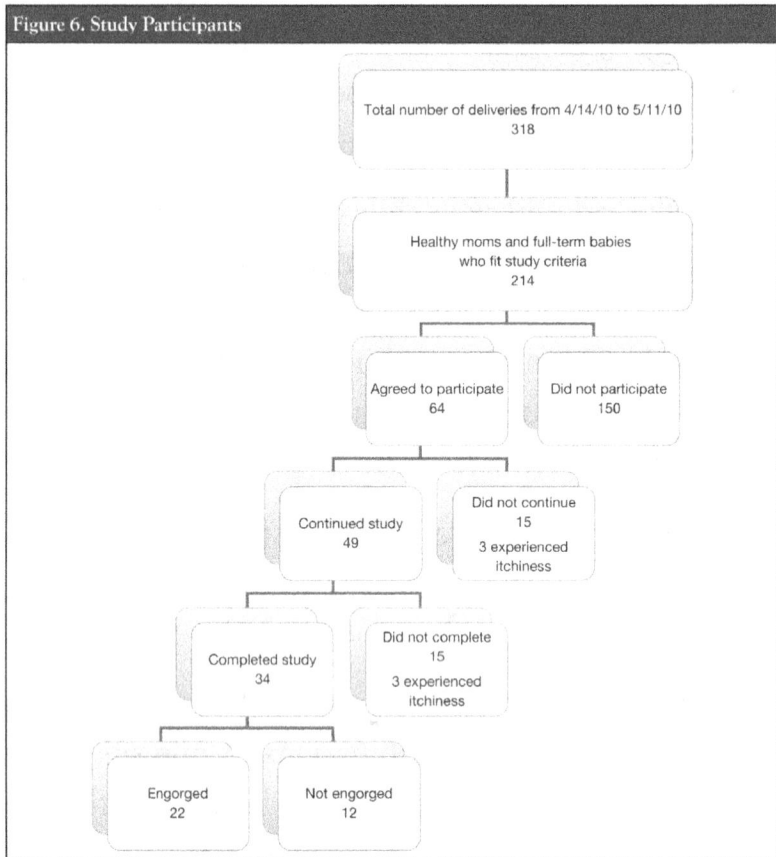

Figure 6. Study Participants

There was no statistically significant difference in engorgement when the entire sample was analyzed using only force gauge measures. We also analyzed force gauge readings as a continuous variable on the subset of the women who were considered engorged by our threshold definition. A paired t-test comparison of untaped versus taped breasts in this subset showed a difference of .148

(95% confidence interval [.017, .279]), but this difference was lower than .20, the value established in this sample as representing sampling variability.

Engorgement in either breast occurred in 65% of the sample. Table 2 shows the distribution of the incidence, using the combination of measures we took to ascertain engorgement. It should be noted that the table has mutually exclusive categories; women who exceeded the threshold in all three measures are counted separately and are not included in the categories of paired measures.

An additional finding is that 3 of the 64 mothers who initially consented and had a sample of tape applied reported itching in the first 24 hours and opted out of the study. Among the 49 who remained in the study long enough to have one breast taped, 3 more participants stopped the study because of itching, resulting in a 9.4% rate of itching because of the tape.

In all cases, the itching was resolved within a few hours once the tape was removed.

Discussion

This study demonstrated that taping with K-ETT does not affect the incidence of engorgement, and practice in our hospital has not changed.

Engorgement is a complex physiological condition with decreased lymphatic drainage and/or increased interstitial fluid being only partial contributors, and clearly, further research into this area is warranted.

Table 1. Results of Three McNemar's Paired Analyses of 34 Participants' Engorgement by Combinations of at Least Two Measures: Pain, Self-Rated Engorgement, and Firmness

Untaped Breast	Taped Breast	
	Number engorged by pain and firmness	Number not engorged
Number engorged by pain and firmness	5	1
Number not engorged	1	27

Untaped Breast	Taped Breast	
	Number engorged by self-rated engorgement and firmness	Number not engorged
Number engorged by self-rated engorgement and firmness	11	4
Number not engorged	1	18

Untaped Breast	Taped Breast	
	Number engorged by pain and self-rated engorgement	Number not engorged
Number engorged by pain and self-rated engorgement	8	1
Number not engorged	4	21

Table 2. Incidence of Engorgement in Either Breast Among 34 Postpartum Women by Combinations of at Least Two Measures: Self-Rated Pain, Self-Rated Engorgement, and Firmness

Measure	Number Engorged	Percentage
Pain and firmness	0	0
Self-rated engorgement and pain	6	18
Self-rated engorgement and firmness	9	26
Pain, self-rated engorgement, and firmness	7	21
Total with engorgement	22	65

Note. Engorgement by pain was any one measure 3 points above baseline, by self-rated engorgement was any measure of 3 or higher, and by firmness was any durometer measure of .20 or higher above baseline. The final determination of engorgement was exceeding these thresholds in at least two of the measures taken.

Our findings related to the overall incidence of engorgement are consistent with many other published reports (ABM, 2009; Hill & Humenick, 1994). There is, however, no widely accepted measure for engorgement, which makes comparisons with other studies difficult.

The pain and self-rated engorgement scales are both subjective, and many mothers seemed not able to distinguish between sources of pain (e.g., nipple pain vs. engorgement pain) or localized differences between their two breasts.

Use of the 6-point engorgement scale (which includes both firmness and pain), but scored by palpation and questioning by a lactation consultant or clinician experienced in evaluating engorgement by palpation, could improve both the validity and reliability of this measure. The durometer or force gauge is a promising tool for objectively measuring the degree of breast firmness, which characterizes breast engorgement.

For future studies, we recommend continued use of the force gauge device, the researcher scoring the engorgement scale, and daily measurements to more closely monitor breast changes. But returning for objective measurements was a hardship for many new mothers, and as a result, a small number of subjects completed our study.

We further recommend in future studies that daily contact with the researcher be done in the mother's home. In addition, a major variable we did not control for was when measurements were made relative to the infant's breastfeeding. Typically, there is a noticeable difference in breast engorgement pre- and post-breastfeeding. In the future, all measurements should be made consistently, either immediately before or after a breastfeeding.

As clinicians working with mothers who develop this self-limited, but difficult, problem, we hope this pioneering study sparks interest to do further research. We need to better understand the physiological process of engorgement and to identify effective preventive and treatment measures for engorgement in postpartum women.

References

Academy of Breastfeeding Medicine Protocol Committee. (2009). ABM clinical protocol #20: Engorgement. *Breastfeeding Medicine*, 4(2), 111–113.

Bourbonnais, F. (1981). Pain assessment: Development of a tool for the nurse and the patient. *Journal of Advanced Nursing, 6*, 277–282.

Chikly, B. (1999, August). *Lymph drainage therapy: Treatment for engorgement.* Paper presented at International Lactation consultant Association (ILCA) Conference, Scottsdale, AZ.

Cotterman, K. J. (2004). Reverse pressure softening: A simple tool to prepare areola for easier latching during engorgement. *Journal of Human Lactation, 20,* 227–237.

Glantz, S. (1997). *Primer of biostatistics* (4th ed.). New York, NY: McGraw-Hill.

Hill, P. D., & Humenick, S. S. (1994). The occurrence of breast engorgement. *Journal of Human Lactation, 10*(2), 79–86.

Kase, K., & Stockheimer, K. R. (2006). *Kinesio Taping® for lymphoedema and chronic swelling.* Albuquerque, NM: Kinesio Taping Association.

Koul, R., Dufan, T., Russell, C., Guenther, W., Nugent, Z., Sun, X., & Cooke, A. L. (2007). Efficacy of complete decongestive therapy and manual lymphatic drainage on treatment-related lymphedema in breast cancer. *International Journal of Radiation Oncology and Biological Physics, 67*(3), 841–846.

Mangesi, L., & Dowswell, T. (2010). *Treatments for breast engorgement during lactation (Review). The Cochrane Library,* (9), CD006946.

Newton, M. & Newton, N. (1951). Postpartum engorgement of the breast. *American Journal of Obstetrics & Gynecology, 61,* 664–667.

Riordan, J. R., & Wambach, K. (2010). *Breastfeeding and human lactation* (4th ed.). Sudbury, MA: Jones & Bartlett Learning.

Roberts, K. L. (1999). Reliability and validity of an instrument to measure tissue hardness in breasts. *Australian Journal of Advanced Nursing, 16*(2), 19–23.

Shim, Y. U., Lee, H. R., & Lee, D. C. (2003). The use of elastic adhesive tape to promote lymphatic flow in the rabbit hind leg. *Yonsei Medical Journal, 44*(6), 1045–1052.

Stamp, G. E., & Casanove, H. T. (2006). A breastfeeding study in a rural population in South Australia. *Rural Remote Health, 495,* 1–8.

Thelen, M. D., Dauber, J. A., & Stoneman, P. D. (2008). The clinical efficacy of kinesio tape for shoulder pain: A randomized, double-blinded, clinical trial. *Journal of Orthopedic and Sports Physical Therapy, 38*(7), 389–395.

Tsai, H. J., Hung, H. C., Yang, J. L., Huang, C. S., & Tsauo, J. Y. (2009). Could Kinesio tape replace the bandage in decongestive lymphatic therapy for breast-cancer-related lymphedema? A pilot study. *Supportive Care for Cancer, 17*(11), 1353–1360.

Yoshida, A., & Kahanov, L. (2007). The effect of kinesio taping on lower trunk range of motions. *Research in Sports Medicine, 15*(2), 103–112.

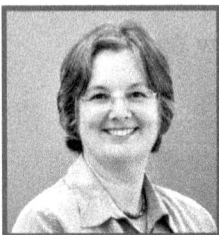

Donna Brown, RN, IBCLC, RLC, CKTP, has worked as a registered nurse in the nursery and NICU in a large San Francisco Bay area hospital for 32 years. She co-founded the lactation services department, and has been working as a lactation consultant for the past 16 years. Donna is a certified Kinesio tape practitioner and hopes to use this skill to make breastfeeding more successful for mothers.

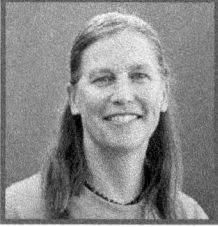

Claire Langdon, MA, RN, IBCLC, RLC, received her master's degree in Zoology from University of California, Berkeley. She worked for 12 years as a research biologist, including being part of the team using recombinant DNA technology to clone interferon. In 1991, Claire retrained as a registered nurse so she could have a more personal impact in women's health, becoming a CLE (UCLA) in 1993, and becoming an IBCLC in 2000.

USLCA

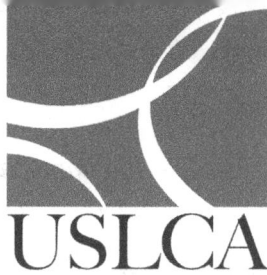

Six Reasons Why Mary Fischer Hated Breastfeeding

(and Six Things I Wish We Could Have Said)

Kathleen Kendall Tackett, PhD, IBCLC, FAPA[1]

Keywords: Nipple pain, breastfeeding, postpartum adjustment

The story of Mary Fischer is a chronicle of what can go wrong in a breastfeeding dyad if the mother receives no skilled lactation help. Mary's downhill slide seemed to start with sore nipples, possibly due to poor positioning. It led to a classic pattern of pain, possibly low milk supply (the baby was "on" all the time), and a mother who was clearly overwhelmed. Unfortunately, this mother was willing to blog about her negative experience, further perpetuating the idea that breastfeeding is a painful and overwhelming act. Her experience could has been so different if she had

1   kkendallt@gmail.com

had the help she needed. It's important for lactation consultants to understand the subjective side of a negative experience, often due to breast or nipple pain, and to realize what a difference they make for the mothers that they do assist.

I was recently surfing my way through social media and I happened upon a blog post entitled *Six Reasons I Hated Breastfeeding and Would Never Do It Again.* I didn't post her article on my Facebook page, but I wanted to hear more about her experience. She breastfed for two weeks and then stopped. And she didn't just hate breastfeeding—she *loathed it.* I wondered why. Why hadn't things worked out for her? How could we have supported her better?

In many ways, Mary's experience highlights the problems that new mothers encounter in the U.S. If we want to prevent premature weaning, we need to listen to women who decide to wean and find out what happened to them once they left the hospital.

The following are Mary Fischer's reasons for why she hated breastfeeding. I think we would hear similar stories from other new mothers.

1. **It's all I did—OMG.** Mary noted that her baby took an hour to feed and the baby was on her 24/7. It was overwhelming.

2. **I needed sleep.** Nighttime feedings also overwhelmed her. It helped when her husband could handle some of these.

3. *It hurt like hell.* Breastfeeding hurt and was making her cry—and she was already crying a lot.

4. *My baby was hungry.* She worried that her baby wasn't getting enough to eat and was fussy as a result. She reported that his demeanor completely changed once he was bottle-fed and had a full belly.

5. *It made me feel more isolated.* Breastfeeding in public was out of the question for her. She felt like she couldn't go out and was very isolated and lonely.

6. *I wanted my body back.* After being pregnant for so many months, she was happier once she had her body back.

Mary has outlined some common reasons mothers cite for why they stop breastfeeding.

The following is what I wish we could have said to Mary before she got to that point.

1. Based on the history Mary reported in her blog post, most of us would recognize that something was not working with her latch. It hurt, but the baby was *all the time,* and the mother reported that her baby seemed hungry. If her baby was gaining well, we could have reassured her and talked with her about how to tell if her baby was getting enough. If I were to see her, my immediate goal would be to address her nipple pain. Something clearly wasn't working and I would want to make sure to address her pain *tout sweet.*

2. Mary Fischer was clearly overwhelmed with the demands of new motherhood. And should we be surprised by her reaction? No! Generally speaking, our culture does an extremely poor job of supporting new mothers. Mothers leave the hospital and step right back in their lives. Rather than having lots of good support from people who come and bring them food, tidy their houses, and sit and talk with them, American mothers are expected to do all the things they normally do plus be up making snacks for everyone who comes to see the baby. No wonder she felt *tied down* by having to hold her baby all the time. She was expected to be *doing something productive* with her time. What could be more productive than what she was already doing? Yet she seemed to feel that she needed to do *more*. When she couldn't meet our society's unrealistic expectations, she felt like she was failing.

3. On a related point, we often do a poor job of preparing mothers for the realities of parenting a baby. Postpartum is hard. It is intense. But it doesn't last forever. Helping mothers to understand that holding the baby is a way to transition him from womb to world often makes it more tolerable. Suzanne Colson explains to mothers that the baby has just come from an environment where he was *held* in utero 24/7. It's not unreasonable for a baby to want to be held a lot as they transition to life outside the womb.

4. It's not hard to understand why she felt so isolated. Unfortunately, we still live in a culture where it is not always safe to nurse a baby in public. The thought of being out and about and still needing to nurse can be a significant barrier for many new mothers. It only takes hearing about one mother forced off a plane, or asked to leave a restaurant, for many other new mothers to decide that they will not risk it. As a result, many women start bottle-feeding because they are finally *broken* by the social isolation. Remember, social isolation is often used as a form of *torture*. It is not surprising that mothers cannot endure it. And they really shouldn't have to.

5. Mary Fischer had also reached her breaking point regarding sleep. The fact that breastfeeding hurt would be enough to keep her from sleeping. If we had been able to address that issue, she would have gotten *more* rest while breastfeeding. Sleep deprivation is also another form of *torture,* and painful breastfeeding was definitely adding to her sleeplessness. It doesn't have to be this way either—nor should it have been.

6. As a final point, we shouldn't overlook the role of postpartum depression in her experience. Mary's pain, sleep problems, and social isolation are practically a recipe for depression. She notes this herself,

> But then when [breastfeeding] pretty much took over my life and made me even more

exhausted, overwhelmed, and depressed than I already was, I realized that breastfeeding was never going to be my cup of tea.

If you've ever have a day where you've wondered if the work you do makes a difference, please remember Mary's story. If not for your efforts, there would be thousands of other mothers who would report a similar tale.

Instead, you help mothers every day get the best possible start to parenting by modeling compassion and providing skilled care. You make a tremendous difference in the lives of the families you serve. Thanks for all you do. And Mary, I'm sorry we failed you. I hope that next time around, you get the support and help you deserve.

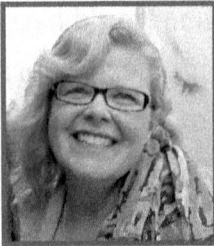

Kathleen Kendall-Tackett, PhD, IBCLC, RLC, FAPA, is a health psychologist, IBCLC, and Fellow of the American Psychological Association. Dr. Kendall-Tackett is Editor-in-Chief of *Clinical Lactation*, clinical associate professor of pediatrics at Texas Tech University Health Sciences Center, and owner of Praeclarus Press www.PraeclarusPress.com.

USLCA

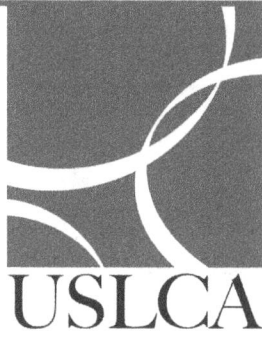

USLCA is a non-profit membership association focused on advancing the International Board Certified Lactation Consultant (IBCLC) in the United States through leadership, advocacy, professional development, and research.

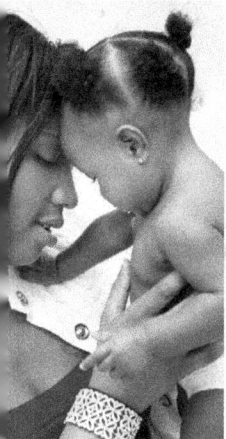

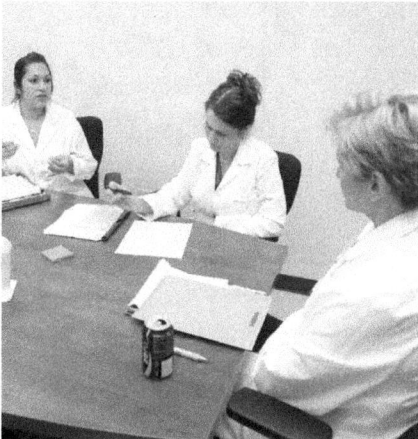

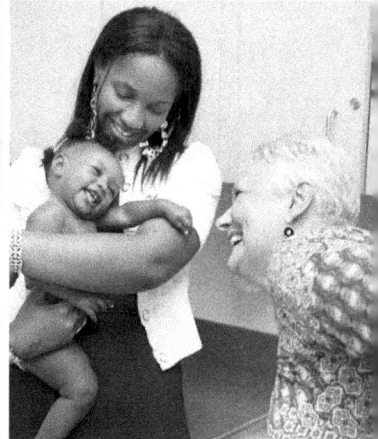

Join USLCA today
202-738-1125 | Washington, D.C. | www.USLCA.org

The U.S. Lactation Consultant Association Presents
Clinical Lactation Monographs

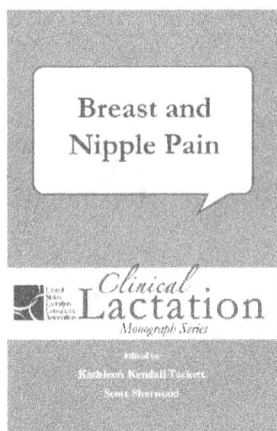

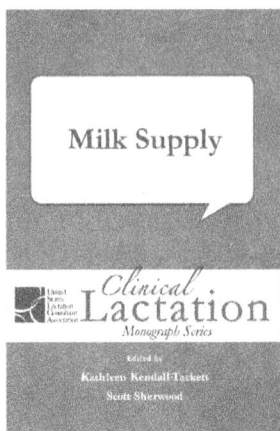

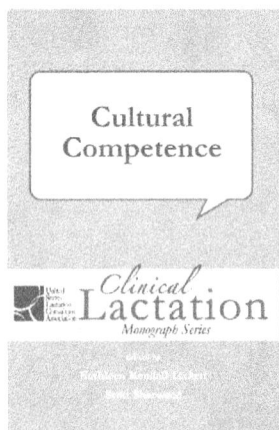

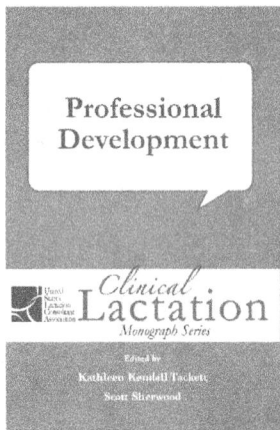

Praeclarus Press
Excellence in Women's Health

www.PraeclarusPress.com

Breastfeeding Titles from Praeclarus Press

Praeclarus Press
Excellence in Women's Health

www.PraeclarusPress.com

www.ingramcontent.com/pod-product-compliance
Lightning Source LLC
Chambersburg PA
CBHW060857280326
41934CB00007B/1089